MUSCLE MASTERY

Your Ultimate Fitness and Nutrition Log Book

Comprehensive Catalogue Of Supplement Guide ♦ *90- Days Fitness Tracker* ♦ *A Series Of Exercise Regimens Spanning 24 Weeks* ♦ *Nutrition And Supplementation Program*

Powered by

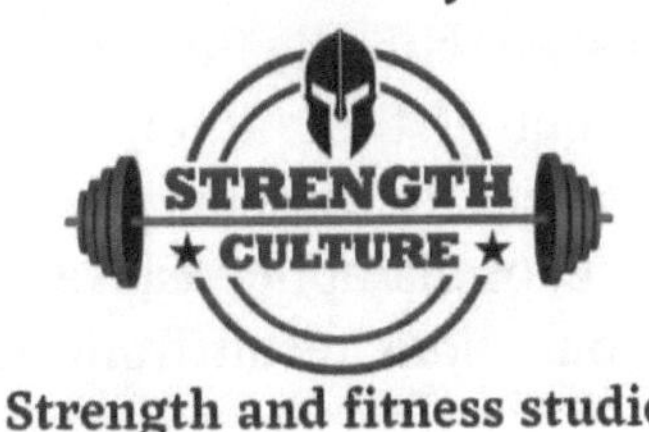

Strength and fitness studio

14/6 North madha church,square lane,
royapuram ,chennai- 600013

+91 9344208650
+91 9790925968

Reach out to us –

Instagram – Fayaz_coach

Gmail – faizu2509@gmail.com

NAME   – ___________________________

PHONE   – ___________________________

EMAIL   – ___________________________

MOHAMMED FAYAZ

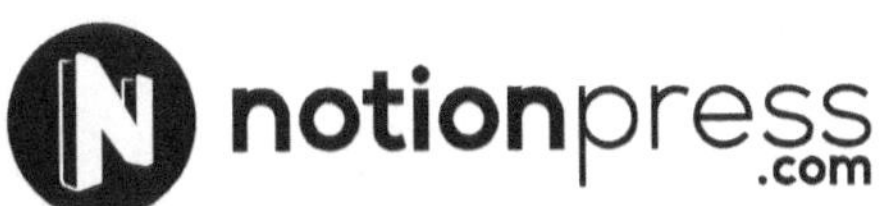

INDIA • SINGAPORE • MALAYSIA

Disclaimer

Table of Contents

Acknowledgement

I would like to express my heartfelt gratitude to the following individuals and organizations who have been instrumental in the creation of this Fitness and Nutrition Log Book:

My dedicated trainer, whose expertise and motivation have guided me on my fitness journey.

My family and friends, for their unwavering support and encouragement throughout my pursuit of a healthier lifestyle.

The fitness community, for inspiring me to push my limits and strive for continuous improvement.

The readers of this log book, whose commitment to health and wellness serves as a constant source of motivation.

Your support and encouragement have been invaluable in shaping this log book and empowering me to stay committed to my fitness and nutrition goals. Thank you for being a part of this journey towards a healthier and happier life.

With gratitude,

Mohammed Fayaz.

CONSISTENCY IS KEY...
KEEP PUSHING YOUR LIMITS...

If an expensive gym membership isn't in your budget, opt for a more affordable one and put in the effort to see results. However, when it comes to nutrition, you can't out-exercise a poor diet. Quality food does come at a higher price. If you can't afford it, don't expect cheaper alternatives to yield the same results. Instead, aim to improve your financial situation to prioritize good nutrition. Remember, staying healthy might be costly, but so are medical bills. Choose your expenses wisely.

– Mohammed Fayaz

Why Did I Write This Book?

The aim of this book is not to turn you into a bodybuilder, provide the ultimate diet plan, or make you superhuman. Instead, the goal is to enhance your understanding of supplementation alongside proper nutrition. We will explore the deficiencies many people face, why relying solely on food may not meet your individual needs, and the crucial role of supplementation, especially for vegans, busy professionals, athletes, women's health and so on. Additionally, we will delve into how supplements can play a vital role in your daily life, improving overall well-being and addressing specific health concerns. Through this book, you will gain the knowledge needed to make informed decisions about your nutritional intake and supplementation for a healthier, more balanced life.

1. FAQ-Why take supplements instead of eating natural foods to fulfill your needs?

While natural foods are essential for a balanced diet, there are several reasons why supplements might be necessary to fulfill your nutritional needs:

- **Nutrient Deficiencies:** Even with a well-balanced diet, some people may still face nutrient deficiencies due to many factors such as soil depletion, food processing, and cooking methods that can reduce the nutrient content in foods.
- **Bioavailability:** Certain nutrients are better absorbed by the body in supplement form. For instance, vitamin B12 and vitamin D are more easily absorbed from supplements than from some food sources, especially for people with specific dietary restrictions or health conditions.

- **Dietary Restrictions**: Vegans, vegetarians, and people with food allergies or intolerances might find it challenging to get all essential nutrients from their diet alone. Supplements can help fill these gaps and ensure they meet their nutritional needs.
- **Health Conditions**: Some health issues or drugs can interfere with nutrient absorption, making it necessary to take supplements to maintain optimal health.
- **Life Stages**: Different life stages, such as pregnancy, breastfeeding, aging, and intense physical activity, require increased nutrient intake. Supplements can help meet these increased demands.
- **Convenience**: In today's fast-paced world we live in, it can be difficult to consistently prepare and consume nutrient-rich meals. Supplements provide a convenient way to ensure you are getting essential vitamins and minerals daily.
- **Environmental Factors**: The body's need for nutrients can be elevated by pollution, stress, and other environmental factors. Using supplements can lessen the effect of these factors on your health.

By understanding these reasons, you can make informed decisions about incorporating supplements into your diet to promote your overall well-being and address specific health concerns.

2. What are some common food adulterations?

Food adulteration involves adding or substituting substances in food items to increase quantity and reduce costs, often compromising safety and quality. Some common forms of food adulteration include:

1. **Addition of Water**: Adding water to milk, which reduces its nutritional value.
2. **Use of Synthetic Colors**: Using harmful synthetic dyes to enhance the appearance of foods like sweets, spices, and beverages.
3. **Adulteration of Oils**: Mixing cheaper oils with more expensive ones, such as adding palm oil to olive oil.

4. **Addition of Starch or Flour**: Adding starch or flour to dairy products like cheese and cream to increase volume.

5. **Contamination with Non-edible Substances**: Adding items like chalk powder to flour, brick powder to chili powder, and sand to sugar to increase weight.

6. **Use of Preservatives**: Adding excessive or banned preservatives to prolong shelf life, such as formalin in fish and fruits.

7. **Artificial Ripening**: Using chemicals like calcium carbide to ripen fruits quickly, which can be harmful to health.

8. **Dilution with Water or Other Liquids**: Diluting juices, honey, and alcohol with water or other liquids to increase volume.

9. **Presence of Pesticides and Chemicals**: Residues from pesticides and chemicals used in agriculture remaining on fruits, vegetables, and grains.

10. **Mislabeling or False Claims**: Labeling products as organic or natural when they are not, misleading consumers.

How to Protect Yourself from Food Adulteration

- **Buy from Trusted Sources**: Purchase food items from reputable vendors and brands.
- **Check for Quality Seals**: Look for certifications from trusted organizations indicating quality and safety standards.
- **Inspect Food Items**: Examine food items for unusual color, texture, or smell.
- **Wash and Peel**: Thoroughly wash fruits and vegetables and peel them if necessary to remove surface contaminants.
- **Stay Informed**: Keep up-to-date with reports from food safety authorities regarding adulteration and recalls.

Being cautious and informed can help reduce the risks associated with food adulteration.

3. What are some common forms of adulteration in the supplement industry and how can consumers protect themselves from these risks?

Adulteration in the supplement industry is a significant concern and can pose serious health risks. Common forms of adulteration include:

1. **Undeclared Ingredients**: Supplements may contain ingredients not listed on the label, such as pharmaceuticals, steroids, or other substances that can cause harm or interact negatively with other medications.

2. **Substitution with Cheaper Ingredients**: Manufacturers may replace expensive active ingredients with cheaper, less effective, or even harmful alternatives. For example, herbal supplements might contain fillers like rice powder instead of the advertised herb.

3. **Incorrect Dosage**: Supplements might not contain the amount of active ingredient stated on the label, leading to underdosing or overdosing, both of which can be dangerous, especially for potent ingredients.

4. **Contaminants**: Supplements may be contaminated with harmful substances such as heavy metals (lead, mercury, cadmium), pesticides, or microbial contaminants due to poor manufacturing practices.

5. **Synthetic Substitutes**: Natural ingredients may be replaced with synthetic versions, which can have different effects and may not be as safe or effective as the natural counterparts.

6. **Use of Banned Substances**: Some supplements have been found to contain substances banned by regulatory agencies due to their potential health risks, such as ephedra or certain anabolic steroids.

7. **False Claims and Mislabeling**: Supplements might be marketed with false claims about their efficacy or benefits, misleading consumers about what they are purchasing.

8. **Inadequate Quality Control**: Poor manufacturing processes can lead to inconsistent product quality, with some batches being pure and others adulterated.

How to Protect Yourself

- **Buy from Reputable Sources**: Purchase supplements from well-known and trusted brands or retailers.
- **Look for Certification**: Check for third-party testing and certification labels (e.g., NSF, USP, FSSAI, ConsumerLab).
- **Check for Recalls and Warnings**: Stay informed about product recalls and warnings from regulatory bodies like the FDA.
- **Consult Healthcare Professionals**: Before taking any supplement, especially if you have underlying health conditions or are taking other medications, consult with a healthcare provider.

Awareness and vigilance can help mitigate the risks associated with supplement adulteration.

Why Track Progress?

"In the journey towards fitness and improved nutrition, tracking progress serves as a compass guiding us towards our goals. It provides tangible evidence of our efforts, revealing what's working and what needs adjustment. By meticulously recording our workouts, dietary intake, and overall progress, we gain invaluable insights into our strengths and weaknesses. This data empowers us to make informed decisions, optimizing our routines for maximum efficiency and results. Moreover, tracking progress fosters accountability, holding us accountable to ourselves and our aspirations. Seeing tangible evidence of progress, whether it's weight loss, muscle gain, or improved performance, fuels motivation and reinforces our commitment to our health journey. Ultimately, a fitness and nutrition log book serves as a personal roadmap, charting our course towards a healthier, stronger, and more vibrant lifestyle."

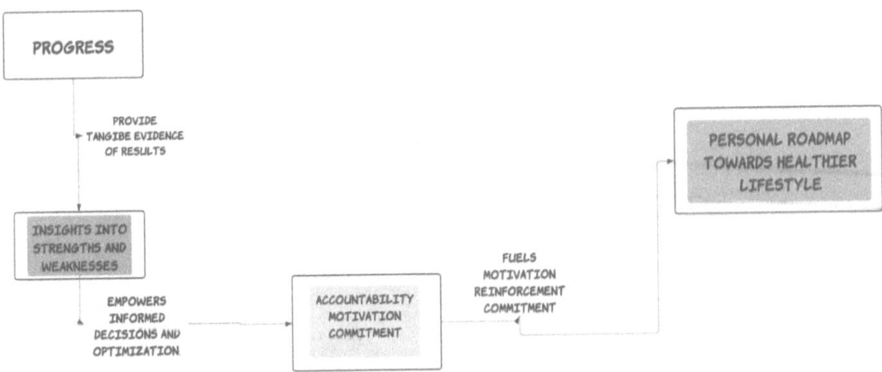

"Fitness is not about being better than someone else. It's about being better than you used to be."

Introduction

Venturing into a fitness journey is not just about physical transformation; it's about embracing a lifestyle that nurtures your body, mind, and spirit. Every journey begins with a single step, and yours starts here. Welcome to the beginning of a transformative experience that will redefine your limits and elevate your well-being.

Starting a fitness journey involves making a commitment to yourself, a promise to prioritize your health and vitality. It's about setting goals that resonate with your aspirations and values, whether it's shedding excess weight, sculpting your physique, improving strength and endurance, or simply enhancing your overall quality of life.

But beyond the tangible outcomes, a fitness journey explores deep self-discovery and individual development. It's about uncovering your inner resilience, pushing past obstacles, and embracing the journey of self-improvement with courage and determination.

As you embark on this adventure, remember that progress is not linear, and challenges are inevitable. But it's in overcoming these challenges that you'll discover your true strength and resilience. Along the way, you'll find a community group of people with similar interests who will provide encouragement and motivation, sharing in your triumphs and lifting you up during moments of doubt.

So, take that first step with confidence, knowing that every effort you invest in yourself helps you get closer to realizing your full potential. Embrace the journey, celebrate your achievements, always keep in mind the amazing potential that exists within you and never let it slip away. Your fitness journey starts now, and the possibilities are limitless.

Preparation for Your Fitness and Nutrition Journey

1. Set Specific, Measurable Goals

- Make sure to establish your fitness objectives, whether they involve losing weight, gaining muscle, improving endurance, or overall health.
- Make your goals specific and measurable, such as "lose 10 lbs. in 3 months" or "run a 5K in under 30 minutes."
- Remember to set both immediate and future objectives to maintain your motivation throughout your journey.

2. Assess Your Current Fitness Level

- Evaluate your current physical abilities, such as strength, flexibility, and cardiovascular fitness.
- Consider taking baseline measurements like weight, body composition, and fitness test results.
- This will help you track your progress and make informed decisions about your fitness plan.

3. Create a Realistic Plan

- Create a well-rounded fitness program that encompasses a variety of components, including a nutritious diet.
- Begin your exercise routine at a moderate pace and gradually escalate the intensity and length of your workouts over time to avoid injury.
- Include various types of exercises in your workout regimen to challenge and develop various muscle groups throughout your body and improve overall fitness.

4. Prioritize Consistency

- Recognize that regularity and persistence are essential elements in attaining and maintaining your desired level of physical fitness.

- Commit to a regular exercise schedule, even if it's just 30 minutes a day.
- Find ways to make fitness a habit, such as scheduling workouts in your calendar or finding a workout buddy.

5. Prepare Mentally

- Acknowledge that your fitness journey will have ups and downs, and be prepared to overcome challenges.
- Cultivate a positive mindset and focus on the progress you're making rather than the setbacks.
- Acknowledge and take pride in your incremental accomplishments throughout your fitness journey to remain motivated and encouraged.

6. Gather Necessary Equipment

- Invest in appropriate workout gear, such as comfortable shoes, breathable clothing, and any necessary equipment for your chosen activities.
- Ensure you have access to the necessary resources, such as a gym membership or home workout equipment.

By taking the time to prepare thoroughly, you'll be well on your way to a successful and sustainable fitness journey.

"Your body will be around a lot longer than the expensive handbag, Invest in yourself "
- unknown.

Nutrition

Nutrition is the vital process through which organisms acquire and utilize nutrients from food to facilitate growth, development, and general well-being. It entails comprehending the significance of diverse nutrients in the body and making informed decisions regarding dietary intake to enhance health. Food sustains the body by delivering crucial nutrients like carbohydrates, proteins, fats, vitamins, minerals, and water. These nutrients play diverse roles, such as fueling energy production, aiding in tissue growth and repair, regulating metabolism, and sustaining overall health.

It's important to eat good foods rather than bad foods because:

- **Nutrient Density:** Good foods are typically nutrient-dense, meaning they provide a high concentration of valuable nutrients relative to their calorie content. In contrast, bad foods often contain excessive calories, processed sugar, unhealthy fats, and additives with little nutritional value.
- **Health Impact:** Eating nutrient-rich foods promotes overall health and lowers the likelihood of chronic conditions like heart disease, diabetes, obesity, and specific cancers. Conversely, poor dietary choices can lead to adverse health effects and elevate the risk of developing such diseases.
- **Energy and Vitality:** Good foods provide the body with high energy and nutrients it needs to function optimally, leading to increased energy levels, vitality, and overall well-being. In contrast, bad foods can lead to fatigue, sluggishness, and poor physical and mental performance.
- **Long-Term Health:** Consistently eating a balanced diet of good foods promotes long-term health and longevity, while consuming

bad foods regularly can have detrimental effects on health and quality of life.

Divisions in nutrition include:

- **Macronutrients:** These are nutrients required in large amounts by the body and include carbohydrates, proteins, and fats. They provide energy and support various physiological functions.
- **Micronutrients:** These are nutrients required in smaller amounts but are essential for various metabolic processes and overall health. Micronutrients include vitamins and minerals.
- **Water:** While not a nutrient in the traditional sense, water is vital for hydration, nutrient transport, temperature regulation, and overall physiological function.

Understanding the principles of good nutrition and making healthy food choices are essential for promoting optimal health, vitality, and longevity.

Let's Talk about Supplements

WHY WE NEED SUPPLEMENTS? IS IT COMPULSORY

Nutritional supplementation involves the act of ingesting dietary supplements, which are designed to complement the diet by supplying essential nutrients that may be deficient or insufficiently consumed through food alone. These supplements can include vitamins, minerals, amino acids, fatty acids, herbal extracts, enzymes, and other substances. The purpose of nutritional supplementation is to fill nutrient gaps, support overall health, and address specific nutritional needs or deficiencies. While balanced, rich whole foods are the foundation of good health, supplements can be used to complement dietary intake, especially when certain nutrients are difficult to acquire in adequate amounts from

food alone or when increased demands exist due to factors like age, lifestyle, or health conditions.

It's important to note that while supplements can play an important role in supporting health, they are not a substitute for a healthy diet and lifestyle. Additionally, the use of supplements should be taken with caution, and help from a healthcare provider is advisable to ensure safety, appropriateness, and effectiveness, particularly for individuals with specific health conditions or those taking medications.

Supplementation is a very interesting field – some people become over-dependent on supplements, and others quickly dismiss the entire concept. The truth is that, done intelligently, supplementation can help address multiple deficiencies in your diet. Based on your health goals, it can be a great, targeted help.

DISCLAIMER – Supplements that are given in the list for every goals should not be consumed without any consultation, the goal of taking supplements is fill the nutritional gaps that are missing from whole foods, which are considered to be quite essential for health (e.g. – vitamin d, b12 etc.) so before your consider taking supplements please get a complete blood work and get to know your deficiencies before you start considering supplements.

Also, please read the detailed information on each and every supplement to know about the right dosage, timing, physiology and impact on health, which are given in the supplementary section.

NOTE – Please refer to the supplement section to learn about the different types, timing, usage, and details of each supplement before starting your supplement regimen.

SUPPLEMENTS FOR GENERAL HEALTH

- Whey protein or plant protein or lean protein foods
- Fish oil or foods containing good fats
- Vitamin D or vitamin D fortified foods
- Zinc
- Magnesium
- Vitamin C
- calcium

RECOMMENDED SUPPLEMENTS

- Fish oil or foods containing good fats
- Vitamin D or vitamin D fortified foods
- Zinc
- Magnesium
- calcium

Taking supplements for general health is not compulsory except for a few and should not replace whole foods. While supplements can provide essential nutrients, they're intended to complement a balanced diet, not substitute it entirely. Whole foods offer a complex plenty of important nutrients, such as vitamins, minerals, fiber, and

phytonutrients that work synergistically to support overall health and well-being. While supplements may fill nutrient gaps in some cases, they lack the diverse array of compounds found in whole foods that contribute to optimal health. Furthermore, relying solely on supplements can lead to nutritional imbalances and may not provide the same benefits as consuming a varied diet rich in fruits, veggies, whole grains, lean proteins, and healthy fats. Therefore, it's essential to prioritize whole foods as the foundation of a healthy diet, using supplements only when necessary and under the guidance of a healthcare professional.

SUPPLEMENTS FOR BODYBUILDING AND STRENGTH

- Whey protein or plant protein or lean protein foods
- Creatine
- Fish oil or foods containing good fats
- Caffeine
- Vitamin D or vitamin D fortified foods
- GDA
- Magnesium
- Zinc
- Calcium
- Taurine
- Glutamine
- Citrulline malate (use only if you have any additional endurance goals)

- **Beta-alanine (use** only if you have any additional endurance goals**)**

RECOMMENDED SUPPLEMENTS

- **Whey protein or plant protein or lean protein foods** (Highly recommended)
- **Creatine** (Highly recommended)
- **Zinc** (Highly recommended)
- **Fish oil or foods containing good fats** (Highly recommended)
- **Vitamin D or vitamin D fortified foods** (Highly recommended)
- **Magnesium** (Highly recommended)
- **Calcium** (Highly recommended)
- **Caffeine (**Use caffeine strategically if you're a very busy professional who demands peak performance in the gym or during physical activities, and you need to maintain your energy levels without experiencing fatigue too quickly**)**
- **Glutamine (**only if you are dealing with gut health issues due to intake of high protein or need a little more additional muscle recovery and digestion**)**
- **Taurine (**only if you are looking to enhance performance and promote greater muscle recovery**)**
- **GDA (**use only if you are in a seriously high-carbohydrate intake, read the supplement section to know more**)**

Supplements for bodybuilding and strength training aren't mandatory but offer benefits. Protein supplements and amino acids aid muscle growth, while creatine supports recovery and enhances strength. Pre-workout supplements provide energy and focus during workouts. They're convenient for busy lifestyles, ensuring essential nutrient intake. Some supplements also promote overall health, which is vital for optimal performance. However, they should complement a balanced diet and training plan, not replace them. Not all supplements are safe or effective, and individual responses vary. Thorough investigation and consultation with healthcare professionals are necessary before supplementing, ensuring reputable brands and evidence-based ingredients.

SUPPLEMENTS FOR WOMEN'S HEALTH

- Whey protein or plant protein or lean protein foods
- Fish oil or foods containing good fats
- Vitamin D or vitamin D fortified foods
- Magnesium
- Zinc
- Myo-inositol
- Calcium
- Iron
- Folic acid
- Probiotics

RECOMMENDED SUPPLEMENTS

- Whey protein or plant protein or lean protein foods
- Fish oil
- Vitamin D or vitamin D fortified foods (Highly recommended)
- Magnesium (Highly recommended)
- Myo-inositol
- Zinc (Highly recommended)
- Calcium (Highly recommended)
- Iron (Highly recommended)
- Folic acid

Top 3 reasons why women need to take supplements:

9. Women tend to have lower muscle mass compared to men, which means they burn fewer calories. Additionally, many women have smaller appetites than men, leading to lower overall caloric

intake. This combination can contribute to nutrient deficiencies, as they may not be consuming enough nutrients to support their bodily needs.

10. Women typically experience menstruation every 28 to 35 days, with individual variations. During this period, they lose blood and experience cramps and mood swings, which also leads to iron loss. To mitigate the risk of iron deficiency, it is crucial for women to supplement with iron and magnesium to maintain optimal iron levels and to get relief from cramps and inflammation also promotes other benefits.

11. Some women experience hormonal imbalance, which can affect their metabolism and lead to conditions like polycystic ovary syndrome (PCOS). PCOS is an endocrine disorder characterized by irregular menstrual cycles, cysts on the ovaries, and insulin resistance. Supplements like myo-inositol can help alleviate these symptoms by promoting hormonal balance, improving insulin sensitivity, and regulating menstrual cycles.

Although supplements can be useful for addressing specific nutritional needs or health concerns, they're intended to complement a balanced diet, not serve as a substitute for nutrient-rich foods. Whole foods offer a variety of important nutrients, including vitamins, minerals, antioxidants, and fiber, that work synergistically to support women's health and well-being. However, certain supplements, such as folic acid during pregnancy or vitamin D for bone health, may be advised in addition to a healthy diet to meet specific nutritional needs. The benefits of taking supplements for women's health include addressing nutrient deficiencies, supporting reproductive health, promoting bone density, and enhancing overall wellness. It's essential to choose supplements wisely, opt for reputable brands with evidence-based ingredients, and get guidance from a healthcare provider before adding any supplement regimen to ensure safety and effectiveness.

SUPPLEMENTS FOR FAT LOSS

- Whey protein or plant protein or lean protein foods
- Fish oil or foods containing good fats
- Vitamin D or vitamin D fortified foods
- Magnesium
- Zinc
- Glutamine
- Caffeine
- Calcium
- Probiotics
- Creatine
- L-carnitine

RECOMMENDED SUPPLEMENTS

- Whey protein or plant protein or lean protein foods
- Fish oil or foods containing good fats (Highly recommended)
- Creatine (use only if you are serious about maintaining muscle mass)
- Vitamin D or vitamin D fortified foods (Highly recommended)
- Magnesium (Highly recommended)
- Zinc (Highly recommended)
- Calcium (Highly recommended)
- Glutamine (use only if protein intake is high and for gut & muscle recovery)
- Caffeine (It's a stimulant, helps in performance, and also creates a thermic effect inside the system, which means it increases resting energy expenditure by a certain degree by using fat as energy. Also, it has few drawbacks, so use it with precaution)
- L-carnitine (L-carnitine is a great choice if you want to use fat as energy by transporting fatty acids into mitochondria; also, if you are a morning person, taking l-carnitine before a workout helps in higher metabolism and promotes performance; read more about this in supplement section)

Due to calorie restriction (less food intake), supplementation does come in very handy during fat loss as it helps in fulfilling the nutrients that are missing from the whole foods which helps in maintaining overall health and for optimal performance.

SUPPLEMENTS FOR GUT HEALTH

- Fish oil or foods containing good fats
- Whey protein
- Digestive enzymes
- Probiotics
- L-glutamine

RECOMMENDED SUPPLEMENTS

Use only if you are dealing with any intolerances or gut issues. Do seek advice from a health care professional before starting any supplements for gut health. Follow a low-FODMAP diet which is available in google before starting with gut health supplements.

- Digestive enzymes
- Probiotics
- L-glutamine
- Fiber (Add soluble and insoluble fiber-rich foods into your diet, which helps gut health and digestion)

Supplementing for gut health can be beneficial for individuals experiencing digestive issues or imbalances in gut bacteria. Probiotics, prebiotics, digestive enzymes, fiber, and gut-healing nutrients are commonly used supplements to support gut health. Probiotics introduce beneficial bacteria to the gut, while prebiotics nourish these bacteria. Digestive enzymes aid in food breakdown, and fiber promotes regular bowel movements and supports the growth of beneficial bacteria. Nutrients like zinc, glutamine, and vitamin A help maintain gut integrity.

These supplements may improve digestion, nutrient absorption, and immune function, as well as reduce symptoms of digestive disorders such as bloating and constipation.

SUPPLEMENTS FOR TESTOSTERONE

- Fish oil or foods containing good fats
- Whey protein or plant protein or lean protein foods
- Ashwagandha
- Boron
- Zinc
- Vitamin D or vitamin D fortified foods
- Magnesium

RECOMMENDED SUPPLEMENTS

Supplements are not the ideal way to increase testosterone unless you are dealing with hormonal issues, low energy, under medication or any other factors. If you are a healthy person, increasing testosterone comes with 3 important things.

- Physical activity
- Eating right nutrition (foods rich in good fats and antioxidants)
- Overall lifestyle

Supplements like vitamin D, boron, zinc, and ashwagandha do come in handy in promoting testosterone. But they are not the replacement for a poor diet and lifestyle.

SUPPLEMENTS FOR BUSY PROFESSIONALS

- Fish oil or foods containing good fats
- Whey protein or plant protein or lean protein foods
- Ashwagandha

- Vitamin D or vitamin D fortified foods
- Melatonin
- Probiotics
- Collagen
- Magnesium
- Zinc

RECOMMENDED SUPPLEMENTS

- **Fish oil or foods containing good fats**
- **Whey protein or plant protein or lean protein foods**
- **Ashwagandha** (Helps relieve stress)
- **Vitamin D or vitamin D fortified foods**
- **Melatonin** (Only if dealing with sleep issues; read more about melatonin in the supplement section)
- **Magnesium**
- **Collagen** (Collagen supplements are a great addition to your daily routine, as they may help support skin, hair, joint health, and overall well-being. If you have a desk job and are frequently exposed to digital devices, you may be more susceptible to issues like hair loss, thinning, or dull skin. In such cases, incorporating collagen supplements into your regimen could help maintain your health and address these concerns)
- **Pre & probiotics** (Only if you are dealing with indigestion, bloating, gas and other gut issues)

Based on the information found, the following are the search results provided. The key recommendations for supplements that can benefit people working in IT or office jobs: These are highly recommended supplements, which are listed below (highly recommended).

Vitamin D: Office workers who spend most of their time indoors are often deficient in vitamin D, which is crucial for supporting healthy bones and the immune system and also enhances overall health and wellness. Aim for at least 3,000 IU of vitamin D per day.

Iron: Iron is crucial for building red blood cells and preventing anemia, which can cause fatigue. Office workers may be at risk of iron deficiency and should consider an iron supplement.

Multivitamin: A high-quality multivitamin can help bridge the nutritional gaps in the diet of busy office workers who may not have time for balanced meals.

Melatonin: For office workers who have trouble falling asleep at night, a melatonin supplement can help regulate the sleep-wake cycle.

Ashwagandha or other adaptogenic herbs: These herbs can aid the body in adapting and managing stress, which is common for those working in high-pressure office environments.

SUPPLEMENTS FOR HAIR, SKIN, JOINTS, SLEEP

Begin by trying any two supplements from the list below, each targeting different goals, and observe any changes or improvements. If you don't notice any positive effects, consider adding different supplements or consult a professional for guidance on addressing the issue.

For example – If you are taking biotin and collagen to improve hair health but experience sleep issues due to stress or other reasons, consider adding melatonin to your routine to address the sleep problem. Observe any changes and improvements.

HAIR

- BIOTIN (Recommended)
- WHEY PROTEIN or PROTEIN-RICH FOODS (Recommended)
- COLLAGEN (REFER TO SUPPLEMENT SECTION) (Recommended)
- VITAMIN C & E
- ZINC (Recommended)
- Fish oil or foods containing good fats

- ASHWAGANDHA (ONLY IF LACK OF SLEEP OR STRESS)
- MELATONIN (ONLY IF LACK OF SLEEP OR STRESS)

SKIN

- COLLAGEN (Recommended)
- VITAMIN C & E (Recommended)
- FISH OIL (Recommended)
- PRE & PROBIOTICS (Recommended)
- ZINC
- GLUTATHIONE

JOINTS

- GLUCOSAMINE & CHONDROITIN (Recommended)
- CALCIUM (Recommended)
- Vitamin D or vitamin D fortified foods (Recommended)
- BORON (Recommended)
- MAGNESIUM (Recommended)
- PROTEIN
- FISH OIL
- TURMERIC

SLEEP

- MELATONIN
- MAGNESIUM (Recommended)
- ASHWAGANDHA
- GLYCINE (Recommended)

Don't start any supplement regimen for sleep if your sleep is a mess. Try to avoid using cell phones or any devices with blue light at least one hour before bed. Make your room pitch black, and avoid drinking any caffeinated beverages within six hours before bedtime. Instead, consider taking a walk or having a warm bath, which might help induce sleep for some individuals. Reading books or practicing breathing exercises can also improve sleep quality. If none of these methods work, you can start with glycine, which is safe and effective for improving sleep. Alternatively, melatonin can be used as indicated in the supplement section. Always seek help from a professional to identify the underlying causes of your sleep issues.

SUPPLEMENTS FOR VEGANS AND VEGETARIANS

- Fish oil or foods containing good fats
- Whey protein or plant protein or pea protein
- Ashwagandha
- Vitamin D or vitamin D fortified foods (Recommended)
- Vitamin-b12 (Recommended)
- Zinc (Recommended)
- Magnesium (Recommended)
- Taurine (Recommended)
- Creatine (Recommended)
- L-carnitine
- Iron (Recommended)

Supplements are essential for vegans and vegetarians to address potential nutrient deficiencies resulting from the exclusion of animal-derived foods. Key nutrients like vitamin B12, omega-3 fatty acids, iron, calcium, and vitamin D may be lacking in plant-based diets. Supplements fill these gaps, supporting overall health, preventing deficiencies, and reducing the risk of chronic diseases. They ensure optimal intake of essential nutrients vital for bone health, immune function, cognitive health, and energy metabolism. By supplementing strategically alongside a balanced plant-based diet, vegans and vegetarians can thrive and enjoy the associated health benefits.

WHY VEGANS AND VEGETARIANS SHOULD TAKE SUPPLEMENTS:

Vegans and vegetarians may face several anti-nutrients in their diets, which can affect nutrient absorption and overall health. Here are some common anti-nutrients and their sources.

- **Phytates:** Found in whole grains, seeds, and legumes, phytates can bind to minerals like zinc, calcium, magnesium, and iron, reducing their absorption.
- **Lectins:** Present in legumes, whole grains, and nuts, lectins can disturb the absorption of calcium, iron, phosphorus, and zinc.
- **Oxalates:** Found in green leafy vegetables, tea, beans, nuts, and beets, oxalates can bind to calcium and prevent its absorption, potentially leading to kidney stone issues.
- **Glucosinolates and Goitrogens:** Present in cruciferous vegetables like broccoli, Brussels sprouts, cabbage, and kale, these compounds can prevent the absorption of iodine, potentially interfering with thyroid function.
- **Saponins:** Found in legumes, saponins can interfere with absorbing minerals and leading to digestive problems.
- **Tannins:** Present in tea, coffee, and some fruits, tannins can bind to minerals and reduce their absorption.

(For e.g) To minimize the effects of anti-nutrients, vegans and vegetarians can follow these tips: When consuming foods rich in iron and zinc, combine them with foods abundant in vitamin C to enhance absorption.

- Soak legumes before cooking to reduce phytates and lectins.
- Time dairy intake to avoid pairing it with high oxalate foods.
- Purchase dairy products fortified with calcium to ensure adequate calcium intake.
- Consider a multivitamin-mineral supplement with about 100% of the daily recommended dose of nutrients as nutrition insurance.

By following these guidelines and maintaining a balanced and varied diet, vegans and vegetarians can minimize the negative effects of anti-nutrients and ensure optimal nutrient absorption.

WHEY PROTEIN

Whey protein, released from milk during cheese production, is highly considered for its premium quality and well-rounded amino acid composition, which are essential for bodily functions. Its popularity among athletes and fitness enthusiasts stems from its rapid absorption and capacity to support muscle growth and recovery.

Production involves extracting whey from milk after cheese-making, followed by filtration to isolate protein from other components.

Subsequently, the protein is dehydrated into a powdered state

Its benefits include supporting muscle growth, aiding recovery post-exercise, offering convenience for protein intake, and assisting in weight management.

For muscle building, consuming 20-40 grams (multiple times a day) **of 1.6 to 2 grams per kg of body weight; for** fat loss, consuming around **1.8 to 2 grams per kg** of whey protein within an hour post-exercise is advisable. It's beneficial for athletes, those with higher protein needs, and even vegetarians and vegans, with lactose-free options available for those with intolerances or allergies.

When purchasing whey protein, consider the type (concentrate, isolate, or hydrolysate), protein content per serving, ingredients, and certifications ensuring quality and purity.

Whey protein's purposes:

Who benefits from whey protein:

The advantages of whey protein extend beyond mere muscle growth and recovery. Here are some of the key uses of whey protein:

- Whey protein stands out as a rich source of branched-chain amino acids (BCAAs), notably leucine, renowned for its essential role in igniting muscle protein synthesis. Consequently, whey protein emerges as a potent supplement for bolstering muscle growth and recovery, particularly when integrated with resistance training.

- **Post-Workout Recovery:** Intake of whey protein following exercise aids in restoring lost amino acids, facilitating quicker recovery, minimizing muscle soreness, and enhancing overall performance. For those leading hectic lives or finding it challenging to fulfill their protein requirements solely through whole foods, whey protein supplements offer a convenient and effective solution to boost protein intake.

- **Weight Management:** Protein helps in satiation (feeling fuller), meaning it can help reduce appetite and support weight loss or weight maintenance goals. Adding whey protein into a balanced diet can be favorable for anyone looking to manage their weight.

- **Immune System Support:** Whey protein contains immunoglobulins and lactoferrin, which may help boost the immune system and provide additional health benefits.

- **Mood and Well-being:** Some studies suggest that whey protein may have a positive impact on mood and overall well-being, although more research is needed in this area.

By understanding the various uses of whey protein, individuals can make better decisions about incorporating this supplement into their diet and fitness regimen to support their specific goals and needs.

Whey protein can be advantageous for various groups, including:

Athletes and Fitness Enthusiasts: Whey protein aids in muscle recovery, growth, and strength development, making it a valuable supplement for individuals involved in rigorous training.

Individuals with Increased Protein Requirements: Those with elevated protein needs, such as individuals aiming for muscle growth, older adults, or those with specific medical conditions, can benefit from incorporating whey protein into their diet.

Vegetarians and Vegans: While whey protein is milk-derived, plant-based alternatives like pea protein or plant protein to those following a vegetarian or vegan diet.

It is important for individuals with lactose intolerance or dairy allergies to choose lactose-free or dairy-free protein options. Moreover, maintaining a well-rounded diet rich in whole foods alongside whey protein supplementation is crucial for optimal health and performance. Seeking help from a healthcare provider or registered dietitian can assist in identifying individual protein needs and the appropriate utilization of whey protein supplements.

Considerations when purchasing whey protein:

- **Varieties of Whey Protein: Whey is available in three primary forms:** concentrate, isolate, and hydrolysate. The concentrate contains some fat and lactose, isolate has most of the fat and lactose removed, and hydrolysate is pre-digested for easier absorption.
- **Check the Protein Content:** Ensure the whey protein supplement contains around 20-25 grams of protein per serving. This ensures you're obtaining the essential protein needed for muscle growth and recovery.
- **Look for Minimal Additives:** Opt for whey protein powders with minimal additional ingredients. Avoid products with excessive additives, artificial sweeteners, and fillers. Choose products with simple ingredient lists to minimize potential allergens or sensitivities.
- **Check for Certifications:** Look for third-party certifications that guarantee the quality and purity of the whey protein, such as NSF International, FSSAI, company authority code, Informed-Choice, or USP Verified. These certifications signify that the product has undergone testing for contaminants and meets specific quality standards.

- **Check for digestive enzymes:** If you're experiencing lactose intolerance or digestive issues with whey protein, it's beneficial to choose a protein supplement that includes added digestive enzymes. These enzymes aid in the efficient breakdown of proteins, carbohydrates, and fats, promoting smoother digestion.

Take into account extra nutrients and flavor: Certain whey protein powders might include supplementary elements such as creatine or glutamine. Consider whether these additional nutrients align with your fitness goals and dietary needs. Also, choose a product that suits your taste preferences and digestive needs.

- **Amino acid profile labeling:**

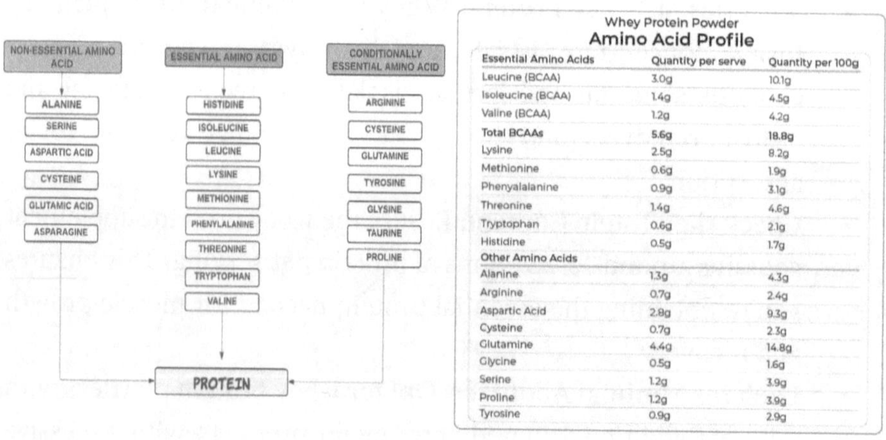

Whey Protein Powder
Amino Acid Profile

Essential Amino Acids	Quantity per serve	Quantity per 100g
Leucine (BCAA)	3.0g	10.1g
Isoleucine (BCAA)	1.4g	4.5g
Valine (BCAA)	1.2g	4.2g
Total BCAAs	5.6g	18.8g
Lysine	2.5g	8.2g
Methionine	0.6g	1.9g
Phenylalanine	0.9g	3.1g
Threonine	1.4g	4.6g
Tryptophan	0.6g	2.1g
Histidine	0.5g	1.7g
Other Amino Acids		
Alanine	1.3g	4.3g
Arginine	0.7g	2.4g
Aspartic Acid	2.8g	9.3g
Cysteine	0.7g	2.3g
Glutamine	4.4g	14.8g
Glycine	0.5g	1.6g
Serine	1.2g	3.9g
Proline	1.2g	3.9g
Tyrosine	0.9g	2.9g

CAFFEINE

Caffeine, a naturally occurring stimulant, is present in multiple plants such as coffee beans, tea leaves, cacao beans (utilized in chocolate production), and kola nuts. It is frequently ingested through beverages like coffee, tea, energy drinks, and certain soft drinks.

Caffeine is also available in supplement form.

How it's Made:

- **Coffee Beans:** Caffeine is taken out from coffee beans through a process of soaking and then separating the caffeine from the beans using a solvent such as water or ethyl acetate.
- **Tea Leaves:** Caffeine is extracted from tea leaves in a similar manner, often using water as a solvent.
- **Synthetic Production:** Synthetically, caffeine can also be manufactured within a laboratory environment.

Uses of Caffeine:

- **Stimulation:** Caffeine is primarily known for its energizing effects on the central nervous system, which can help increase alertness, concentration, and energy levels.
- **Performance Enhancement:** It is commonly used by athletes and fitness enthusiasts to improve exercise performance, endurance, and focus.
- **Fat Loss:** Caffeine supplement is sometimes included in the fat loss phase due to their potential to increase metabolism and fat oxidation.
- **Mental Function:** It may enhance cognitive function, memory, and mood.

Recommended Dosage for Building Muscle:

The optimal dosage of caffeine for muscle building can differ depending on factors such as individual tolerance, body weight, and sensitivity to caffeine. However, research suggests that consuming **1.5-3 mg of caffeine per kilogram** of body weight about 30-60 minutes before exercise may enhance performance and promote muscle strength and power.

Who Should Take Caffeine:

While caffeine can be helpful for many individuals, it's not suitable for everyone. Generally, adults who are not sensitive to caffeine and do not have underlying health conditions that may be exacerbated by its effects can safely consume moderate amounts. However, pregnant women and individuals with cardiovascular issues, anxiety disorders, or sleep disorders should exercise caution or get guidance from a healthcare professional before consuming caffeine.

Impact on Performance:

Caffeine impacts performance through several mechanisms:

- **Stimulation:** Caffeine acts as a stimulant, primarily targeting the central nervous system. Caffeine stimulation can lead to increased feelings of alertness and wakefulness. It has also been demonstrated that caffeine has been shown to reduce the perceived level of effort or exertion during physical exercise. By lowering the perceived difficulty of a workout, caffeine may enable individuals to exercise for longer durations or at higher intensities.
- **Fatigue Delay:** It can delay fatigue by inhibiting the action of adenosine, a neurotransmitter that supports sleep and relaxation.
- **Metabolism:** Caffeine increases metabolism and fat oxidation, potentially providing more energy for exercise.
- **Muscle Contraction:** Caffeine may enhance muscle contraction force and power output.

It's crucial to recognize that people's reactions to caffeine can differ significantly. While moderate consumption is generally safe and may provide benefits like increased alertness, consuming too much caffeine can trigger unpleasant side effects in some individuals. These may include feelings of nervousness or jitteriness, heightened anxiety, difficulty sleeping, or digestive issues such as an upset stomach. It's essential to be mindful of your personal tolerance and adjust your caffeine intake accordingly to avoid these potential negative consequences.

Moderation and awareness of personal tolerance levels are key when using caffeine as a performance enhancer.

When Should I Take Caffeine:

Consume caffeine about **30-60 minutes** prior to your workout to allow enough time for it to be absorbed and reach its maximum concentration in your bloodstream. This timing can help ensure that you experience the performance-enhancing effects of caffeine during your exercise session.

The ideal caffeine dosage may differ based on factors like body weight, tolerance, and individual sensitivity to caffeine. Start with a lower dosage **(e.g., 100-200 mg)** and gradually increase as needed, while being mindful of potential side effects such as jitteriness or insomnia, don't consume any type of caffeine 4 to 6 hours before bed time.

Caffeine recycling:

Caffeine can enhance performance during workouts due to its stimulant properties, but it also has drawbacks, such as slowing down recovery and creating dependency. The time it takes for caffeine to clear from the body varies from **6 to 8 hours**, sometimes longer depending on the dosage, which can hinder post-workout recovery. Furthermore, prolonged use can lead to dependency. To mitigate these issues, it is suggested to cycle caffeine every 30 days or use it only when needed to avoid dependency and support recovery.

FISH OIL

Fish oil is a supplement made from the tissues of oily fish like salmon, mackerel, herring, sardines, and anchovies. It contains high omega-3 fatty acids, especially Alpha-lipoic acid (ALA), eicosapentaenoic acid (EPA) and docosahexaenoic acid (DHA), vital fatty acids known for their various health benefits.

How it's made:

- **Extraction**: Fish oil is typically obtained through molecular distillation, where fish tissues are heated to evaporate the oils and separate them from contaminants like heavy metals and pollutants.
- **Purification**: The extracted oil undergoes purification to remove impurities and ensure its safety and quality.
- **Concentration**: Some fish oil supplements undergo further processing to concentrate the omega-3 fatty acids, increasing their potency per serving.

Uses of Fish Oil:

Fish oil, abundant in omega-3 fatty acids, offers numerous health advantages. These essential fatty acids have demonstrated positive effects on cardiovascular well-being by reducing triglycerides. Lowering blood pressure levels significantly reduces the risk of developing heart disease. Attacks and strokes. Specifically, DHA is pivotal for brain function, enhancing cognitive functions like memory and focusing mood regulation. Additionally, both EPA and DHA possess anti-inflammatory properties that may alleviate symptoms associated with inflammatory conditions like arthritis and inflammatory bowel disease. Interestingly, omega-3 fatty acids also contribute to maintaining healthy eyes and vision, with DHA being an integral retina component.

Recommended Dosage:

While fish oil does not directly contribute to muscle building and strength gains, its anti-inflammatory characteristics can aid in post-exercise recovery and alleviate exercise-induced muscle soreness. The suggested intake of fish oil differs based on individual requirements and health conditions. Typically, consuming approximately **950-1000 milligrams of EPA and DHA (highly recommended) or 500 mg (minimum)** combined daily is recommended for maintaining overall health. However, higher doses may be advised for specific health needs or objectives, underscoring the importance of consulting a healthcare provider for personalized recommendations.

Who Should Take Fish Oil:

"Did you know that fish oil supplements offer a wide range of health benefits?" individuals, including:

- **Those with Cardiovascular Risk Factors:** People with high triglyceride levels, hypertension, or a family history of heart disease may benefit from fish oil supplementation to support heart health.
- **Individuals with Inflammatory Conditions:** Fish oil's anti-inflammatory properties may help alleviate symptoms of conditions such as arthritis, asthma, or inflammatory bowel disease.
- Omega-3 fatty acids are vital for the healthy development of your baby during pregnancy. Development, particularly for brain and eye development in the unborn baby.
- **Athletes and Fitness Enthusiasts:** While not directly linked to muscle building, fish oil may support recovery and overall health in individuals engaged in intense training.

Health Benefits of Fish Oil:

- **Heart Health:** Fish oil supplements have been shown to offer cardiovascular benefits by lowering triglycerides, favorably modifying cholesterol ratios, and reducing blood pressure; all of these factors help lower the risk of heart disease. Moreover, the omega-3 fatty acids present in fish oil are vital for proper brain maturation and cognitive performance, with research suggesting they may help stave off age-related mental decline and enhance emotional well-being.

- **Joint Health:** Fish oil's anti-inflammatory properties may help alleviate arthritis symptoms and improve joint mobility and flexibility.

- **Eye Health:** DHA is a significant retina component, supporting visual development and reducing the risk of age-related macular degeneration.

Impact on Performance:

While fish oil is not a performance-enhancing supplement like protein or creatine, its anti-inflammatory properties may indirectly support exercise performance by reducing exercise-induced inflammation and promoting faster recovery. By minimizing muscle soreness and inflammation, fish oil supplementation may help athletes and fitness enthusiasts maintain training intensity and frequency, leading to better long-term performance outcomes. However, individual responses to fish oil supplementation may vary, and more research is needed to understand its effects on exercise performance fully.

Storage:

Proper storage of fish oil supplements is essential to maintain their quality and prevent them from becoming rancid. Here are some tips for storing fish oil supplements:

- **Cool, Dark Place:** Store fish oil supplements in a cool, dark place to maintain their quality. Avoid placing them in direct sunlight and heat sources. Sources are crucial as exposure to light and heat can accelerate oxidation, leading to the degradation of the supplements.

- **Refrigeration**: Storing fish oil supplements in the refrigerator is essential. However, it can extend their shelf life, mainly if you reside in a warm climate or the supplements have added antioxidants or are liquid.

- **Airtight Container**: Keep fish oil supplements in their original airtight container or an opaque one. Keep them in a tightly sealed container to shield them from contact with air and moisture, which can contribute to oxidation and spoilage.

- **Avoid Humidity**: Moisture can cause fish oil capsules to soften or become sticky, so they should be stored in a dry environment. Avoid storing them in the bathroom or near sources of moisture.

WHEN SHOULD I TAKE FISH OIL:

For better absorption, it is recommended that fish oil supplements be taken with a meal that includes healthy fats, such as omega-3-rich foods like salmon or avocados. This timing helps to enhance the absorption of the omega-3 fatty acids, particularly EPA and DHA, into the bloodstream.

What to look out for when buying fish oil:

- **Omega-3 Content:** "It is known for its omega-3 fatty acid content, specifically EPA (eicosapentaenoic acid) and DHA (docosahexaenoic acid)." Look for the amounts of EPA and DHA per serving on the label. Higher concentrations **(900-1000mg)** are typically better.

- **Purity:** Check for indications of purity and absence of contaminants like mercury, PCBs (polychlorinated biphenyl), and other heavy metals. Labels may mention molecular distillation or other purification methods.

- **Fish Species:** The label should specify the source of the fish oil. Look for reputable fish species like anchovy, sardine, mackerel, or salmon. These incredible species often exhibit lower levels of contaminants and higher concentrations of omega.

CREATINE

Creatine occurs naturally in the body and is present in small quantities in certain foods, especially meat and fish. The human body also produces creatine endogenously, primarily in the liver, kidneys, and pancreas, from amino acids like glycine and arginine. Approximately 95% of the body's total creatine stores are found in skeletal muscle, where it serves as a rapid energy source during high-intensity exercises like weight training and sprinting. The remaining 5% of creatine is distributed in the brain, testes, and other tissues.

How it's Made:

- **Synthesis:** The body primarily produces creatine from the amino acids arginine, glycine, and methionine.
- **Supplementation:** Creatine supplements are typically made by combining creatine monohydrate, the most common form of creatine used in supplements, with other ingredients to form a powder or capsule.

Uses of Creatine:

- **Muscle Building:** Creatine supplementation is widely used. Athletes and bodybuilders commonly utilize creatine supplementation to enhance muscle mass strength and power output, particularly during resistance training.
- **Exercise Performance:** Creatine enhances the body's ability to produce ATP (adenosine triphosphate), the primary energy currency of cells, leading to improved performance during high-intensity, short-duration activities.
- **Recovery:** creatine supplementation has the potential to decrease muscle damage and inflammation after exercise, promoting quicker recovery and reduced muscle soreness.
- **Brain Health:** Research indicates that supplementing with creatine could offer cognitive advantages, potentially enhancing

memory and brain function, especially in individuals with lower creatine levels like vegetarians and vegans.

Recommended Dosage for Muscle Building and Strength:

The standard dosage of creatine for muscle building and strength gains typically involves a loading phase followed by a maintenance phase:

- The typical creatine supplementation protocol involves the loading phase. During the loading phase, it is important to consume **20 grams per day**, split into 4 doses. Equal doses of 5 grams each, taken for **5-7 days.** This loading phase is designed to rapidly saturate the muscles with creatine. However, the loading phase is not mandatory, and some individuals may prefer to skip it to avoid potential side effects like bloating and gastrointestinal discomfort. After the loading phase or for those who do not load, a maintenance dose of **3-5 grams** of creatine per day is recommended to maintain elevated creatine levels in the muscles. More advanced athletes may benefit from a higher maintenance dose of **7-10 grams** per day. Consistent daily intake is crucial to sustain the benefits of creatine supplementation.

Who Should Take Creatine:

Creatine supplementation may be beneficial for various individuals, including:

- **Athletes and Bodybuilders:** Creatine can enhance muscle mass, strength, and exercise performance, making it popular among athletes engaged in high-intensity training.
- **Vegetarians and Vegans:** Since creatine is primarily found in meat and fish, vegetarians and vegans may have lower creatine levels and could benefit from supplementation.
- **Older Adults:** Creatine supplementation may help offset age-related muscle loss and strength decline, improving overall physical function and quality of life.

Who Should Avoid Taking It:

While creatine is generally safe for most people when used as directed, there are some individuals who may want to avoid or use caution with creatine supplementation, including:

- **Those with Kidney Issues:** People with pre-existing kidney conditions or impaired kidney function should use creatine with caution and under medical supervision.
- **Young Adolescents:** While research on the safety of creatine supplementation in adolescents is limited, some experts recommend avoiding creatine use in individuals under the age of 18 due to concerns about potential effects on growth and development.

WHEN SHOULD I TAKE CREATINE?

For better absorption, it is recommended to take creatine shortly after a workout with a combination of lukewarm water and a pinch of salt. This timing allows for optimal muscle creatine uptake and replenishment of depleted creatine stores in the muscle. Creatine is often more soluble in warm fluids, so mixing it with lukewarm water or a warm beverage may help improve its dissolution and absorption.

Sodium can increase the solubility of creatine, potentially making it easier to dissolve and absorb in the digestive tract. This increased solubility may result in faster absorption and utilization by muscle cells.

GLUTAMINE

Glutamine is a non-essential amino acid, meaning your body can produce it naturally. It's the most abundant amino acid found in your muscles and blood. However, during times of stress or intense exercise, your body's demand for glutamine may exceed its ability to produce it, leading to a condition called "conditional essentiality," where it must be obtained through diet or supplementation.

How It's Made:

Glutamine is synthesized in the body from another amino acid called glutamate, with the help of an enzyme called glutamine synthetase. Additionally, it can be taken from dietary sources like protein-rich foods such as meat, fish, dairy products, eggs, and certain vegetables like cabbage, spinach, and beans.

Uses and Dosage:

- **Muscle Building and Strength:** Glutamine is often touted as a supplement to support muscle growth and strength. The typical recommended dosage for muscle-building purposes ranges from **5 to 15 grams per day**, usually taken in divided doses throughout the day.

Who Should Take Glutamine?

- **Athletes and Bodybuilders:** Those engaged in intense physical training may benefit from glutamine supplementation to support muscle recovery and immune function.
- **Individuals with Gastrointestinal Issues:** Glutamine plays an important role in repairing the intestinal lining, which makes it a potentially valuable supplement for individuals dealing with gut issues such as leaky gut, irritable bowel syndrome (IBS), or Crohn's disease.

Who Should Avoid Taking Glutamine?

- **People with Certain Medical Conditions:** Individuals with certain medical conditions such as kidney disease, liver disease, or those prone to seizures should avoid glutamine supplementation unless directed by a healthcare professional.
- **Pregnant or Breastfeeding Women:** Although glutamine is generally a safe supplement to consume, pregnant or nursing women should seek help from a healthcare provider before incorporating any supplements into their routine.

Health Benefits and Gut Health:

- **Gut Health:** Glutamine plays an important role in maintaining and repairing the intestinal mucosa, which is vital for gut health. It's used by intestinal cells as a source of energy and also serves as a precursor for the production of other amino acids and compounds necessary for gut function and repair.
- **Immune Function:** Glutamine is essential for the proper functioning of immune cells and has been shown to support immune function, especially during times of stress or illness.
- **Muscle Recovery:** Glutamine is involved in protein synthesis and can help speed up muscle recovery after intense exercise.

Before initiating any new supplement regimen, particularly if you have any underlying health conditions or concerns, it is crucial to seek guidance from a healthcare provider, as glutamine supplementation may offer benefits for specific individuals.

WHEN SHOULD I TAKE GLUTAMINE?

To enhance the absorption of glutamine, it is recommended to take it about **10-15 minutes** before a meal, ideally on an empty stomach. This helps for better absorption and utilization of the supplement. While it is suggested to take glutamine 2-3 times per day, before 2-3 meals, the key is to ensure consistency in taking it to support gut health and overall well-being.

ZINC

Zinc, an essential mineral vital for immune health, wound healing, and DNA synthesis, is naturally present in foods such as meat, fish, poultry, whole grains, nuts, and legumes. It plays an important role in supporting a strong immune system by increasing the generation of. T-cells, which combat infections.

Uses and Dosage:

- **Uses:** Zinc is commonly used to treat conditions like zinc deficiency, diarrhea, acne, diabetes, and age-related macular degeneration.
- **Dosage for Building Muscle and Strength:** While there is no specific dosage for building muscle and strength, supplementing with 15–30 mg of elemental zinc daily may support overall health, including muscle function.

Effects on Testosterone:

- **Testosterone:** Zinc is linked to testosterone production, and low levels of zinc may lead to reduced testosterone levels. Sufficient zinc consumption is vital for preserving optimal testosterone concentrations, which are necessary for building and maintaining muscular mass and power

Who Should Take Zinc:

- **Who Should Take It:** People following restrictive eating patterns, experiencing impaired nutrient absorption, or having specific medical issues may benefit from zinc supplements. It is especially important for pregnant women to support normal growth and development.

Who Should Avoid Taking Zinc:

- **Who Should Avoid It:** Although zinc is typically safe for the majority of people when consumed in accordance with recommended guidelines, excessive zinc intake can lead to toxicity. Individuals with certain medical conditions like Wilson's disease should avoid zinc supplements unless prescribed by a healthcare provider.

Health Benefits and Women's Health:

- **Health Benefits:** Zinc has anti-inflammatory properties that are beneficial for skin health, wound repair, and immune function. It may help with conditions like acne, rosacea, psoriasis, and eczema.
- **Women's Health:** Zinc supports normal growth and development during pregnancy and is essential for overall health. Adequate zinc intake is crucial for women to maintain immune function, skin health, and overall well-being.

In conclusion, zinc is a vital mineral with diverse health benefits, including supporting muscle function, immune health, and skin health. It is essential for individuals aiming to build muscle and strength, but it is important to follow recommended dosages and seek help from a healthcare provider before starting any supplementation regimen.

WHEN TO TAKE ZINC FOR BETTER ABSORPTION?

To optimize the absorption of zinc, it is recommended to take the supplement either an hour before a meal or two hours after eating. This timing is crucial because certain nutrients, like fiber and some minerals, can interfere with zinc absorption. In case zinc supplements lead to stomach discomfort, they can be consumed alongside a meal, but spacing them apart from iron or calcium supplements is important to avoid interference with absorption. Additionally, acidic foods like vinegar and those rich in vitamin C can support zinc absorption. Zinc is most bioavailable from animal sources, and for vegetarians and vegans, it's essential to be mindful of phytates in plant foods that can hinder zinc absorption.

GLUCOSE DISPOSAL AGENT (GDA)

GDA, or Glucose Disposal Agent, is a type of dietary supplement designed to enhance the body's ability to manage and utilize glucose effectively. GDA typically contains a combination of ingredients such as herbs, minerals, and vitamins that are believed to support glucose metabolism.

How It's Made:

GDA supplements are typically formulated using a combination of ingredients that have been shown to influence glucose metabolism. Common ingredients may include chromium picolinate, alpha-lipoic acid, cinnamon extract, berberine, and bitter melon extract, among others.

Effect on Health:

The purported effects of GDA supplements include:

- **Enhanced Glucose Uptake:** GDA supplements are believed to improve the uptake of glucose by muscle cells, which may enhance energy production during exercise and support muscle growth and recovery.
- **Insulin Sensitivity:** Certain components in GDA supplements are believed to enhance insulin sensitivity, enabling cells to better respond to insulin and manage blood sugar levels.

Dosage:

Dosage recommendations for GDA supplements can vary depending on the specific formulation and ingredients. Adhering to the manufacturer's guidelines or seeking personalized guidance from a healthcare professional is crucial.

Who Should Take GDA?

- **Athletes and Bodybuilders:** Individuals looking to optimize their nutrient partitioning and support muscle growth and recovery may consider using GDA supplements as part of their supplementation regimen.
- **Those with Blood Sugar Concerns:** People with concerns about blood sugar regulation or insulin sensitivity may find GDA supplements beneficial, although they should consult with a healthcare professional before use.

Who Should Avoid Taking GDA?

- **Individuals with Medical Conditions:** Individuals with specific health issues, including diabetes or metabolic disorders, should refrain from using GDA supplements unless directed by a healthcare professional, as they may interfere with medication or exacerbate existing health issues.
- **Pregnant or Breastfeeding Women:** The safety of GDA supplements during pregnancy and breastfeeding has not been well studied, so it's advisable for pregnant or breastfeeding women to avoid them.

Health Benefits and Gut Health:

- **Blood Sugar Management:** GDA supplements can aid in maintaining optimal blood sugar levels and enhancing insulin sensitivity, which is important for overall metabolic well-being
- **Muscle Building and Strength:** By promoting glucose uptake into muscle cells, GDA supplements may support muscle growth and strength gains, especially when combined with resistance training.
- **Gut Health:** Some ingredients in GDA supplements, such as cinnamon extract and berberine, have been studied for their potential benefits for gut health, including anti-inflammatory and antimicrobial effects.

Although GDA supplements could provide advantages for specific individuals, it is crucial to approach their use with care and seek help from a healthcare provider before initiating any new supplement routine, particularly if you have existing health issues or uncertainties. Furthermore, prioritizing a well-rounded diet and consistent physical activity continues to be fundamental for overall well-being and physical fitness.

WHEN SHOULD I TAKE GDA?

Take GDA supplements approximately 15 to 30 minutes before consuming a high-carbohydrate meal. This timing allows the ingredients in the supplement to begin working before you ingest carbohydrates, enhancing glucose disposal and utilization.

Take GDA supplements with your largest meals of the day, especially those containing a significant amount of carbohydrates. This ensures that the supplement is utilized when your body needs it most to manage glucose levels effectively.

VITAMIN D (cholecalciferol)

Vitamin D is an extremely important nutrient required for optimal bodily function. It helps keep our bones strong, our immune system healthy, and our muscles working well. It also makes us feel good overall. Vitamin D helps the body absorb calcium, which is essential for maintaining strong bones. It also has properties that reduce inflammation in our body.

Vitamin D (sun exposure) Fair vs dark skin:

The skin has the ability to produce vitamin D when exposed to sunlight, particularly ultraviolet B (UVB) radiation. It is also available from sources like fatty fish (e.g., salmon and mackerel), fortified foods (e.g., milk, orange juice, cereals), and supplements. Vitamin D absorption from sunlight is influenced by skin pigmentation, with fair-skinned individuals generally able to produce more vitamin D than those with darker skin. This difference is attributed to the varying levels of melanin in the skin, which affects the efficiency of ultraviolet B (UVB) radiation in stimulating vitamin D synthesis. Fair-skinned individuals with lower melanin levels can produce vitamin D more effectively due to the increased penetration of UVB radiation into their skin. This allows them to generate sufficient vitamin D with relatively shorter periods of sun exposure, typically around 15 minutes. In contrast, darker-skinned individuals. Individuals with greater melanin concentrations are less able to generate vitamin D from sun exposure. This is because melanin absorbs and scatters UVB radiation, making it less effective in stimulating vitamin D synthesis. As a result, darker-skinned individuals require longer periods of sun exposure, typically around 30 to 40 minutes, to achieve the same level of vitamin D production. These differences in vitamin D absorption from sunlight are crucial for maintaining optimal vitamin D levels, which are extremely important for various body functions, such as bone health, immune system, and overall health.

Effect on Health:

- **Bone Health:** Vitamin D is necessary for calcium absorption and bone mineralization, which are essential to keep bones strong and avoid issues such as osteoporosis.
- **Immune Function:** Vitamin D plays a role in modulating immune function and may help reduce the risk of certain infections and autoimmune diseases.
- **Muscle Function:** Having sufficient vitamin D levels is linked to enhanced muscle strength and performance, which can positively impact athletic abilities and overall movement.

Dosage:

- The suggested daily amount of vitamin D differs based on factors like age, gender, and personal requirements.
- For adults, the recommended dietary allowance (RDA) is typically around **2000-4000 IU per day.**
- Some research recommends that higher doses of vitamin D, up to **5000 IU per day**, may benefit muscle health and strength, especially in individuals with low vitamin D levels.
- To boost vitamin D levels fast for those who do not get enough exposure to sunlight or are deficient in vitamin D and calcium absorption, taking vitamin D **(60000 IU) once a week for 12 weeks** can help boost vitamin D levels.

Health Benefits and Gut Health:

- **Immune Support:** Having sufficient vitamin D levels is linked to a lower likelihood of respiratory infections and can aid in improving overall immune function.
- **Cardiovascular Health:** Vitamin D might offer protective benefits for heart health by reducing the chances of heart disease and enhancing the regulation of blood pressure.

- **Gut Health:** Vitamin D receptors are found throughout the gastrointestinal tract, and vitamin D may play a role in maintaining gut barrier function and modulating the gut microbiome.

Timing for Better Absorption:

Vitamin D supplements, being fat-soluble, can be better absorbed when consumed with a meal that includes dietary fat. Some studies propose that taking vitamin D supplements with the main meal of the day could improve absorption, as the fat content in the meal aids in the absorption of fat-soluble vitamins.

Consultation:

- Seeking help from a healthcare professional is crucial before initiating any new supplement regimen, including vitamin D supplementation, especially if you have underlying health conditions or are taking medications.
- A health professional can assist in determining the suitable dosage of vitamin D tailored to your specific requirements and health condition.

By ensuring adequate vitamin D intake through sunlight exposure, dietary sources, or supplementation, you can support muscle health, strength, and overall well-being.

VITAMIN-B12 (COBALAMIN)

Vitamin B12, which is also called cobalamin, is a type of water-soluble vitamin. is indispensable for the proper functioning of the human body. It is extremely important for maintaining healthy nerve tissue, facilitating DNA production, and enabling the formation of the metabolism of red blood cells, fats, proteins, and carbohydrates.

Vitamin B12 is made by bacteria living in animals' intestines, including humans. However, the human body cannot produce vitamin B12 on its own, so it must be obtained through dietary sources or supplements.

In the body, vitamin B12 is primarily absorbed in the small intestine, particularly in the ileum, with the help of a protein called intrinsic factor, which is produced by the stomach. Without intrinsic factors, the body cannot effectively absorb vitamin B12 from food or supplements, which can lead to a deficiency.

Certain groups of people are at a higher risk of vitamin B12 deficiency and may benefit from supplementation. These include:

- **Vegans and vegetarians:** Due to the fact that vitamin B12 is predominantly present in animal-derived foods, individuals who follow a vegan or vegetarian may not obtain adequate amounts solely through their dietary choices.
- **Older adults:** As individuals progress in age, their bodies may experience a decline in the efficiency of absorbing vitamin B12 from dietary sources.
- **Individuals with gastrointestinal disorders:** Conditions such as Crohn's disease, celiac disease, and atrophic gastritis can affect the absorption of vitamin B12.
- **Those who have had weight loss surgery:** Certain medical procedures, such as gastric bypass surgery, can diminish the body's capacity to effectively absorb vitamin B12.

- **People with pernicious anemia:** This autoimmune condition affects intrinsic factor production, leading to impaired vitamin B12 absorption.

Timing:

The timing of vitamin B12 supplementation isn't as critical as ensuring consistent intake. However, some people find it easier to remember to take their supplements at a specific time, such as with breakfast or dinner.

The best form of B12 can vary based on individual genetics and needs. There are three main types of B12 that are considered beneficial: **hydroxocobalamin, methylcobalamin, and adenosylcobalamin.** The recommended dosage varies depending on age, dietary habits, and individual needs. It's essential to follow the instructions on the supplement label or seek help from a healthcare professional for personalized advice.

When choosing a B12 supplement, it's crucial to consider factors like absorption rates and stability. Cyanocobalamin, the most common form found in supplements, has low absorption rates and requires conversion into hydroxocobalamin before the body can utilize it effectively. On the other hand, **methylcobalamin** is considered more bioavailable and remains in the body for longer periods, supporting liver, brain, and nervous system health. **Methylcobalamin** is also known for its role in improving visual accommodation, modulating melatonin secretion, and reducing homocysteine levels, which is beneficial for cardiovascular health.

Dosage:

Adult men & women – 2.4 micrograms per day
Pregnancy – 2.6 micrograms per day
Lactation – 2.8 micrograms per day
Kids (age 9-13) – 1.8 microgram per day

MAGNESIUM

Magnesium occurs naturally in the Earth's crust and is present in a variety of foods, such as leafy greens and nuts, seeds, whole grains, and some types of fish. It's also commonly found in mineral-rich water sources.

The body benefits from magnesium supplementation in several ways:

- **Supporting muscle function:** Magnesium is necessary for proper muscle contraction and relaxation, making it essential for athletes and individuals engaging in physical activity.
- **Promoting nerve function:** Magnesium plays a role in regulating the function of neurotransmitters, essential for facilitating communication between nerve cells.
- **Maintaining heart health:** Magnesium is involved in maintaining a steady heartbeat and supporting cardiovascular function.
- **Bone health:** Magnesium works alongside calcium and vitamin D to support bone density and strength.
- **Regulating blood sugar levels:** The involvement of magnesium in insulin metabolism and glucose regulation is significant for individuals managing diabetes or insulin resistance.
- **Sleep:** Magnesium plays an important role in the regulation of neurotransmitters, including gamma-aminobutyric acid (GABA), which is a neurotransmitter known for its soothing effects on the brain, promoting relaxation and facilitating sleep. Additionally, magnesium can help regulate the body's internal clock and promote the production of melatonin, a hormone that regulates sleep-wake cycles. Certain studies indicate that magnesium supplementation may enhance sleep quality and duration, especially in individuals experiencing insomnia or suboptimal sleep quality, particularly in individuals with insomnia or poor sleep quality. However, individual responses

to magnesium supplementation may vary, and more research is needed to fully understand its effects on sleep.

- **Muscle health:** Magnesium is important for proper muscle function, including muscle contraction and relaxation. Magnesium helps regulate calcium ions, which are essential for muscle contraction. A deficiency in magnesium can result in muscle cramps, spasms, and weakness. While magnesium alone may not directly "build" muscle mass like protein or resistance training does, it plays a supportive role in overall muscle health and function. Adequate magnesium levels can help optimize muscle performance and recovery, which may indirectly support muscle growth and maintenance when combined with proper nutrition and exercise.

- **Menstrual Health:** Magnesium may help alleviate symptoms associated with menstruation, such as menstrual cramps (dysmenorrhea) and premenstrual syndrome (PMS). Magnesium's muscle-relaxing properties can help ease muscle tension and reduce the severity of menstrual cramps. Additionally, magnesium supplementation has been shown to potentially reduce the intensity of PMS symptoms, including mood swings, irritability, and bloating.

There are several types of magnesium supplements available, each with slightly different properties:

- **Magnesium oxide:** This form has a high magnesium content but is not well absorbed by the body, making it more likely to cause digestive discomfort like diarrhea.

- **Magnesium citrate:** Magnesium citrate is a form that is more readily absorbed compared to magnesium oxide and is frequently utilized as a laxative owing to its capacity to relax the muscles within the intestines.

- **Magnesium glycinate:** This form is chelated with the amino acid glycine, which enhances absorption and is less likely to cause gastrointestinal side effects.

- **Magnesium chloride:** Typically found in topical formulations like magnesium oil or bath salts, this form can be absorbed through the skin and is sometimes used to alleviate muscle cramps or promote relaxation.

The timing of magnesium supplementation isn't as critical as consistent intake, but some people prefer to take it in the evening to help with relaxation and aid sleep. However, magnesium supplements can be taken with meals to improve absorption, as stomach acid released during digestion helps break down the supplement.

The best form of magnesium ultimately depends on individual needs, preferences, and tolerance. **Magnesium glycinate** is a best form and is recommended for its high absorption rate and minimal gastrointestinal side effects, but other forms may be suitable depending on the intended use and individual response. It is important to seek help with a healthcare professional for personalized advice on magnesium supplementation.

The recommended daily allowance (RDA) for magnesium fluctuates based on factors such as age, gender, and individual health factors. Here are the general guidelines for magnesium intake:

- **Adult Women:** The Recommended Dietary Allowance (RDA) for magnesium for adult women is around **310-320** milligrams per day.
- **Adult Men:** The RDA for magnesium for adult men is slightly higher, around **400-420** milligrams per day.
- **Pregnant Women:** Pregnant women have increased magnesium needs to support fetal growth and development. The RDA for magnesium during pregnancy is around **350-360** milligrams per day.
- **Breastfeeding Women:** Breastfeeding women also require higher levels of magnesium to support lactation. The RDA for magnesium during breastfeeding is around **310-320** milligrams per day.

BORON

Boron is a trace mineral that is naturally present in the environment and found in specific foods, soil, and water sources; it serves diverse functions in the body and is associated with numerous potential health advantages.

Bone Health: Boron, a crucial trace mineral, plays a significant role in maintaining bone health by facilitating calcium, magnesium, and vitamin D metabolism, which is crucial for bone formation and upkeep. Research indicates that supplementing with boron may increase bone density and can help reduce the likelihood of developing osteoporosis.

- **Joint Health:** Boron may have anti-inflammatory properties and could potentially benefit joint health by reducing inflammation and discomfort associated with conditions such as osteoarthritis.
- **Brain Function:** Research has explored the potential impact of Boron on cognitive function and brain health. Some research suggests that boron may help support brain function and cognitive performance, although more studies are needed to fully understand its effects.
- **Wound Healing:** Boron is believed to contribute to the wound healing process by facilitating the production of collagen, a protein essential for tissue repair and regeneration.
- **Hormonal Health:** Boron has been studied for its potential effects on hormone levels, particularly testosterone. Some research suggests that boron supplementation may increase testosterone levels, although results are mixed, and more studies are needed to confirm these effects.

The timing of boron absorption isn't well-established, but taking boron supplements with meals may enhance absorption, as dietary fat can aid in the absorption of fat-soluble nutrients.

As for dosage, there isn't a well-established Recommended Dietary Allowance (RDA) for boron, as it is considered a trace mineral and required in relatively small amounts. Boron supplements commonly offer doses between **6 to 20 milligrams per day**, with the ideal dosage varying based on individual requirements and health circumstances. While boron supplementation may have health advantages, excessive consumption may result in symptoms of toxicity such as nausea. Vomiting, diarrhea, and abdominal discomfort. Hence, it is crucial to adhere to recommended dosages and seek help from a healthcare provider before initiating any new supplement routine, especially if you have pre-existing health conditions or if you are taking medication.

As for who can take boron supplements, they may be suitable for individuals looking to support bone health, joint health, cognitive function, or hormonal balance. However, for pregnant or breastfeeding women, as well as individuals with certain medical conditions or who are taking any medications, it's important to consult with a healthcare professional.

CALCIUM

Calcium, a vital mineral crucial for various physiological functions such as bone formation, muscle activity, nerve signaling, blood clotting, and hormone release, is the most prevalent mineral in the human body, predominantly stored in bones and teeth. Calcium is obtained through dietary sources such as dairy products (milk, cheese, yogurt), leafy greens (kale, broccoli), nuts, seeds, and fortified foods. The body absorbs calcium from the intestines into the bloodstream, which can be utilized for various functions.

Calcium is Widely utilized for maintaining bone health; calcium supplements are commonly used to mitigate or manage calcium deficiency, which may result in conditions like osteoporosis and osteopenia. Here are some potential benefits of calcium supplementation:

1. **Bone Health:** Calcium, a vital constituent of bone tissue, is crucial for constructing and preserving robust and healthy bones. Supplementing calcium may help mitigate bone loss and help lower the risk of fractures, especially in individuals predisposed to osteoporosis or those with insufficient dietary calcium intake.

2. **Muscle and Nerve Function:** Calcium is involved in muscle contraction and nerve transmission, helping muscles contract and relax properly and facilitating communication between nerve cells.

3. **Blood Clotting:** Calcium plays an important role in the blood clotting mechanism, aiding in the formation of blood clots to halt bleeding following an injury

The timing of calcium supplementation is not as crucial as maintaining a consistent intake, but it is generally advised to divide the daily dose into two or more smaller portions taken throughout the day to optimize absorption. Calcium supplements are best absorbed when consumed with food, as stomach acid released during digestion facilitates calcium absorption.

The appropriate daily amount of calcium to consume depends on one's age, sex, and individual health circumstances. The general guidelines for calcium intake are as follows:

- Children 1-3 years: **500 mg/day**
- Children 4-8 years: **700 mg/day**
- Children 9-11 years: **1,000 mg/day**
- Adolescents 12-18 years: **1,300 mg/day**
- Adult Men and Women under 50 years old: **1500-2500** milligrams per day.
- Adult Men and Women over 50 years old: **1500-2000** milligrams per day.

Individuals who may benefit from calcium supplementation include:

- Those with low dietary calcium intake.
- Women who are pregnant or breastfeeding.
- Postmenopausal women at risk of osteoporosis.
- Individuals with conditions that affect calcium absorption, such as lactose intolerance or celiac disease.
- Those who have undergone certain medical procedures, such as gastric bypass surgery.

There are several types of calcium supplements available, including:

- **Calcium carbonate:** Calcium carbonate, the most frequently utilized form of calcium in supplements, relies on stomach acid for absorption and is recommended to be consumed with food for optimal effectiveness.
- **Calcium citrate:** For individuals with low stomach acid levels or those taking acid-reducing medications, calcium citrate is a preferred option due to its high bioavailability, which allows for efficient absorption even in conditions where stomach acid is limited.

- **Calcium gluconate**: Calcium gluconate, a form of calcium primarily used in intravenous (IV) treatments for severe calcium deficiencies, is not commonly found in oral supplements.

When selecting a calcium supplement, it is crucial to choose one that aligns with your specific requirements and preferences. Additionally, it is highly recommended to seek help from a healthcare professional before starting any new supplement routine, particularly if you have existing health issues or are currently taking medications.

IRON

Iron is a mineral essential for various bodily functions, primarily for the production of hemoglobin. It is a protein found in red blood cells that facilitates the transport of oxygen from the lungs to the body's tissues. Iron is also involved in energy metabolism, immune function, and DNA synthesis.

Iron is obtained through dietary sources such as meat, poultry, fish, beans, lentils, spinach, fortified cereals, and grains. The body absorbs iron from the small intestine into the bloodstream, where it is transported to various tissues and organs for use.

Iron supplements are frequently prescribed to manage iron deficiency anemia, a disorder marked by insufficient hemoglobin and red blood cells resulting from inadequate dietary iron intake or absorption. Here are some potential benefits of iron supplementation:

- **Treatment of Iron Deficiency Anemia:** Iron supplements aid in restoring iron reserves within the body and increase hemoglobin levels, improving symptoms such as fatigue, weakness, shortness of breath, and pale skin associated with iron deficiency anemia.
- **Improvement of Exercise Performance:** Sufficient iron levels play an important role in transporting oxygen to muscles during physical activity. Iron supplementation may help improve exercise performance and endurance in individuals with iron deficiency.
- **Support for Cognitive Function:** Iron plays a role in brain development and cognitive function. Iron supplementation may be helpful for individuals with iron deficiency anemia who experience cognitive impairment or poor concentration.

Symptoms of iron deficiency:

Symptoms of low iron levels include tiredness, lack of energy, shortness of breath, difficulty concentrating, frequent illness, pale skin, heart palpitations, headaches, and more. Iron supplements are recommended for individuals experiencing symptoms of iron deficiency, especially those at risk, like pregnant individuals, infants, people with heavy periods, cancer patients, and those with certain health conditions.

Timing:

The timing of iron supplementation can influence absorption. Iron supplements are well absorbed when taken on an empty stomach (recommended), preferably in the morning or between meals, with water or juice containing **vitamin C**, which can enhance iron absorption. However, some people may experience gastrointestinal discomfort when taking iron supplements on an empty stomach, so taking them with food is an alternative option.

The recommended dietary allowance of iron varies depending on age, sex, and individual health factors. Here are the general guidelines for iron intake:

- **Children (male & female) aged 1-3:** 7 milligrams per day
- **Children (male & female) aged 4-8:** 10 milligrams per day
- **Older Kids (male)age 9-13:** 8 milligrams per day
- **Teen (male) age 14-18:** 11 milligrams per day
- **Older Kids (female)age 9-13:** 8 milligrams per day
- **Teen (female) age 14-18:** 15 milligrams per day
- **Adult Men:** 8 milligrams per day
- **Adult Women:** 18 milligrams per day
- **Pregnant Women:** 27 milligrams per day

Types of Iron:

Heme iron (found in animal sources)

Non-heme iron (found in plant sources)

Non-heme iron from plant sources is not the most effective type of iron due to the presence of phytates, oxalates, and tannins, which inhibit iron absorption and result in lower bioavailability compared to heme iron from animal sources. Therefore, if you are vegan or vegetarian, it is advisable to supplement with iron at the recommended dosage to prevent symptoms of anemia, low hemoglobin levels, and low energy.

Iron supplements are typically available in two main forms:

- **Ferrous iron:** This form of iron is more easily absorbed by the body and is found in supplements such as ferrous sulfate, ferrous gluconate, and ferrous fumarate.
- **Ferric iron:** This form of iron is less readily absorbed and is found in supplements such as ferric citrate and ferric sulfate.

Iron supplementation may be beneficial for women's health, particularly during pregnancy and menstruation, when iron needs are increased. Females face an elevated likelihood of iron deficiency due to menstrual blood loss and heightened iron needs during pregnancy to facilitate fetal growth and maturation. Iron supplements may help prevent or treat iron deficiency anemia in women of childbearing age, pregnant women, and breastfeeding mothers. Before initiating any new supplement routine, it is important to seek help from a healthcare professional, as excessive iron consumption can be detrimental, particularly for individuals with specific health conditions or genetic disorders like hemochromatosis.

FOLIC ACID

Folate, also known as folic acid or vitamin B9, is a water-soluble B-complex vitamin that is essential for numerous biological processes in the body. Here's an overview of folic acid, its importance, benefits, impact on gym performance, causes of deficiency, importance for women's health, best time to take it, and dosage:

What is Folic Acid?

Folic acid is the artificial counterpart of folate, a vitamin found naturally in foods such as leafy greens, legumes, and citrus fruits. It is essential for numerous biological processes in the body, including DNA synthesis, cell division, and red blood cell formation.

Importance and Benefits of Folic Acid:

- **DNA Synthesis and Cell Division:** Folic acid is crucial for synthesizing DNA and RNA, which are essential for cell division and growth.
- **Red Blood Cell Formation:** Folic acid plays a vital role in the making of red blood cells, which transport oxygen throughout the body.
- **Prevention of Neural Tube Defects:** Sufficient folic acid intake before and during pregnancy is important for helping neural tube defects, such as spina bifida, in newborns.
- **Heart Health:** Folic acid aids in reducing elevated Homocysteine levels, an amino acid linked with a heightened risk of heart disease when found at elevated concentrations.
- **Brain Function:** Folic acid may support healthy brain function and diminish the risk of age-related cognitive decline.
- **Mood Regulation:** Folic acid plays a vital role in the making of neurotransmitters like serotonin, which regulates mood.

Impact on Performance:

Folic acid indirectly supports gym performance by contributing to overall health and energy metabolism. It aids in red blood cell formation, oxygen transport, and energy production, all of which are essential for physical performance during workouts.

Causes of Folic Acid Deficiency:

Several factors can contribute to folic acid deficiency, including:

- Inadequate dietary intake of folate-rich foods.
- Malabsorption disorders that affect the absorption of nutrients in the intestines.
- Increased demand for folic acid during pregnancy or periods of rapid growth.
- Specific drugs, such as anticonvulsants and methotrexate, may disturb folate absorption.

Women's Health:

Folic acid is particularly important for women's health, especially during pregnancy. Sufficient folic acid intake before conception and during the early stage of pregnancy can greatly decrease the likelihood of neural tube defects in newborns. It also supports overall reproductive health and may help prevent anemia during pregnancy.

Best Time to Take for Better Absorption:

Folic acid supplements can be taken at any time of day, with or without food. However, some studies suggest that taking folic acid supplements with meals may enhance absorption. It's important to adhere to the dosage guidelines provided on the supplement packaging or as directed by a healthcare professional.

Dosage:

The recommended dietary intake of folic acid varies depending on age, gender, and life stage:

- For most adults, including pregnant women, the recommended daily intake is **400 micrograms (mcg)** of folic acid.
- Pregnant women may need higher doses, typically around **600-800 mcg** per day, to support fetal development.
- Individuals with certain medical conditions or those taking medications that interfere with folate absorption may require higher doses under medical supervision.

Before commencing any supplementation regimen, particularly during pregnancy or if you have existing health conditions, it is advisable to consult with a healthcare professional. They can provide tailored advice based on your specific requirements and situation.

Can men take folic acid supplements?

Yes, men can take folic acid, and it can be beneficial for their health as well. While folic acid is often emphasized for its importance in prenatal care and women's health, it also plays an important role in various biological processes in men's bodies. Here are some reasons why men may benefit from folic acid supplementation:

- **Heart Health:** Folic acid aids in reducing elevated homocysteine levels, a condition linked to a heightened risk of cardiovascular disease. By reducing homocysteine levels, folic acid may support heart health in men.
- **Sperm Health:** Folate deficiency has been linked to decreased sperm count and poor sperm quality. Adequate folic acid intake may help improve sperm health and fertility in men.
- **Cognitive Function:** Folic acid plays a vital role in neurotransmitter synthesis and may support cognitive function. Some research suggests that adequate folate levels may aid in lowering the risk of age-related cognitive impairment, including men.
- **Energy Metabolism:** Folic acid is involved in energy metabolism and red blood cell formation, which are essential for overall health and vitality.

- **General Health and Well-Being**: Folic acid supports various bodily functions, including DNA synthesis, cell division, and immune function. Supplementing with folic acid may help maintain overall health and well-being in men.

While men typically require lower doses of folic acid compared to pregnant women, they can still benefit from ensuring adequate intake through diet or supplementation, especially if they have specific health concerns or risk factors. However, it's essential for men to get advice and guidance from a healthcare professional before starting any new supplement regimen to determine their individual needs and ensure proper dosage and safety.

MYO-INOSITOL

Myo-inositol is a naturally occurring compound that belongs to the vitamin B-complex family. It plays an important role in various cellular functions and is particularly important for women's health, reproductive function, and hormonal balance. Here's an overview of myo-inositol, its importance, benefits, impact on gym performance, reasons for use, importance for women's health, best time to take it, and dosage:

What is Myo-Inositol?

Myo-inositol is a type of inositol, which is a group of naturally occurring sugar alcohols that are structurally similar to glucose. It is found in many foods, particularly fruits, grains, and beans, and is also synthesized by the human body.

Importance and Benefits of Myo-Inositol:

- **Hormonal Balance:** Myo-inositol plays a key role in insulin signaling and sensitivity, which helps regulate blood sugar levels and may support hormonal balance, particularly in conditions like polycystic ovary syndrome (PCOS).
- **Reproductive Health:** Myo-inositol supplementation has been shown to improve ovarian function, menstrual regularity, and fertility in women with PCOS. It may also support egg quality and improve pregnancy outcomes.
- **Mood Regulation:** Myo-inositol is involved in the synthesis of neurotransmitters like serotonin, which regulate mood and assist in easing symptoms of anxiety and depression.
- **Supports Skin Health:** Some research suggests that myo-inositol supplementation may improve skin conditions like acne by modulating hormone levels and reducing inflammation.
- **Weight Management:** Myo-inositol may aid in promoting a healthy metabolism and managing weight by enhancing insulin sensitivity and decreasing cravings for carbohydrates.

Impact on Gym Performance:

While myo-inositol is not typically associated with direct effects on gym performance or athletic performance, its role in supporting metabolic health and hormone balance may indirectly contribute to overall energy levels, endurance, and recovery.

Reasons for Use:

Myo-inositol is commonly used as a nutritional supplement for various health purposes, including:

- Supporting hormonal balance and fertility in women with PCOS.
- Managing symptoms of anxiety and depression.
- Improving insulin sensitivity and blood sugar control.
- Supporting skin health and managing acne.

Importance for Women's Health:

Myo-inositol is particularly important for women's health due to its role in reproductive function, hormone regulation, and fertility. It may help improve menstrual regularity, ovulatory function, and fertility outcomes in women with conditions like PCOS.

Best Time for Better Absorption:

Myo-inositol supplements can be taken at any time of day, with or without food. However, some individuals may prefer to take it with meals to enhance absorption. It's important to follow the dosage instructions provided on the supplement packaging or as directed by a healthcare professional.

Dosage:

The recommended dosage of myo-inositol may vary depending on the specific health condition being addressed. For PCOS and fertility support, typical dosages range from **2,000 to 4,000 milligrams (mg)** per day, divided into two or three doses. It is important to discuss with a healthcare professional for tailored guidance based on individual health requirements and circumstances. They can assist in determining the suitable dosage and duration of supplementation for specific health objectives.

Can women supplement with myo-inositol if healthy?

Yes, women can take myo-inositol even if they are healthy. While myo-inositol is often associated with certain health conditions like polycystic ovary syndrome (PCOS) or mood disorders, it can also be beneficial for supporting overall health and well-being in women who do not have these conditions. Here are some reasons why healthy women may consider taking myo-inositol:

- **Hormonal Balance:** Myo-inositol supports hormonal balance by improving insulin sensitivity and signaling. Even in healthy individuals, maintaining stable blood sugar levels and hormonal balance is important for overall health, energy levels, and mood stability.
- **Reproductive Health:** Myo-inositol may support ovarian function, menstrual regularity, and fertility even in women without PCOS or other reproductive health conditions. By promoting healthy ovulation and egg quality, myo-inositol supplementation may help support reproductive health in healthy women as well.
- **Mood Regulation:** Myo-inositol is involved in the synthesis of neurotransmitters like serotonin, which regulate mood. Supplementing with myo-inositol may help support mood stability, minimize symptoms of anxiety and depression, and enhance overall emotional well-being in healthy women.
- **Skin Health:** Some research suggests that myo-inositol supplementation may improve skin conditions like acne by modulating hormone levels and reducing inflammation. Healthy women may benefit from myo-inositol's potential skin-supporting effects, particularly if they experience occasional breakouts or skin issues.

- **Metabolic Health:** Myo-inositol supports metabolic health by improving insulin sensitivity and glucose metabolism. Even in healthy individuals, maintaining optimal metabolic function is vital for overall health, energy levels, and weight management.

It is important to seek advice from a healthcare professional before starting with any new supplements, particularly in case of any pre-existing health conditions or if already on medications, as they can provide tailored plans based on your individual health status and help determine the suitable dosage and duration of supplementation for your specific needs, as myo-inositol is generally considered safe for most individuals.

BIOTIN (VIT B7)

What is Biotin?

Biotin is a coenzyme involved in numerous enzymatic reactions in the body, particularly those related to the metabolism of carbohydrates, fats, and proteins. This process is needed to maintain healthy hair, skin, and nails, as well as aid in energy metabolism and nervous system function, which is important for overall well-being.

Importance and Benefits of Biotin:

Hair, Skin, and Nail Health: Biotin is also known as the "beauty vitamin" due to its ability to enhance healthy hair, skin, and nails. It helps in the making of keratin, a protein that creates the foundation of hair, skin, and nails.

- **Energy Metabolism:** Biotin is involved in the process of carbohydrates, fats, and protein metabolism. It helps convert these nutrients into usable energy for the body.
- **Nervous System Function:** Biotin contributes significantly to the maintenance of nervous system health and may support cognitive function and mood stability.
- **Cell Growth and Repair:** Biotin is necessary for cell growth, repair, and replication, contributing to overall tissue maintenance and regeneration.
- **Pregnancy and Fetal Development:** Biotin is important for fetal development during pregnancy and may support healthy growth and development of the baby.

Impact on Hair Health:

Biotin is often praised as a remedy for hair loss, thinning hair, and enhancing hair growth. While research on the direct effects of biotin supplementation on hair health is limited, biotin deficiency has been linked with hair loss and thinning hair. Supplementing with biotin may help support overall hair health and strength, particularly in individuals with biotin deficiency or certain hair conditions.

Reasons for Use:

People may consider using biotin supplements for various reasons, including:

- Promoting healthy hair, skin, and nails.
- Supporting energy metabolism and vitality.
- Managing symptoms of biotin deficiency, such as hair loss, brittle nails, and skin rashes.
- Supporting overall health and well-being.

Best Time to Take for Better Hair Health:

Biotin supplements can be taken at any time of day, with or without food. However, some people prefer to take them with meals to enhance absorption. There is no specific time of day that is considered best for taking biotin supplements for hair health. Consistency in supplementation is more important than timing.

With Which Foods Should Biotin Be Combined for Better Absorption?

Although biotin supplements are readily available, you can also increase your biotin intake through dietary sources. Foods rich in biotin include:

- Egg yolks
- Liver and other organ meats
- Nuts and seeds (such as peanuts and almonds)
- Legumes (such as beans, lentils)
- Whole grains
- Mushrooms
- Sweet potatoes
- Avocado

Combining biotin-rich foods with a balanced diet can help ensure adequate intake and absorption of this important vitamin. Additionally, consuming foods high in protein and other nutrients that support hair health, such as vitamins A, C, and E, zinc, and omega-3 fatty acids, can further support overall hair health and vitality.

ASHWAGANDHA

What is Ashwagandha?

Ashwagandha, a plant with adaptogenic properties, is native to India and North Africa. It is known for its ability to help the body cope with stress and support overall health and vitality. The roots and flora of the ashwagandha plant are used to make herbal supplements, extracts, and teas.

Importance and Benefits of Ashwagandha:

- **Adaptogenic Properties:** Ashwagandha is categorized as an adaptogenic herb, meaning it assists the body to adapt to the stressors and maintain homeostasis. It may help reduce stress, improve resilience, and enhance overall well-being.
- **Stress Reduction:** Historically, Ashwagandha has been used to reduce stress and anxiety, enhance relaxation, and improve mood.
- **Energy and Vitality:** Ashwagandha may support energy levels, stamina, and physical performance, making it beneficial for athletes and individuals seeking to improve endurance and vitality.
- **Immune Support:** Ashwagandha has immune-modulating properties and may help support immune function and resilience to infections.
- **Brain Health:** Some research suggests that ashwagandha may support cognitive function, memory, and brain health by minimizing oxidative stress and inflammation in the brain.
- **Hormonal Balance:** Ashwagandha may help support hormonal balance and reproductive health in both men and women.

Evidence of Reducing Stress:

Numerous investigations have explored the impact of ashwagandha on stress reduction and anxiety. While more research is needed to fully understand its mechanisms of action and clinical efficacy, preliminary evidence suggests that ashwagandha may help reduce stress and anxiety levels in certain populations, including individuals with generalized anxiety disorder (GAD) and chronic stress.

Reasons for Use:

People may consider using ashwagandha supplements for various reasons, including:

- Managing stress and anxiety
- Supporting overall health and vitality
- Enhancing physical and mental performance
- Promoting relaxation and sleep quality

Importance for Overall Health:

Ashwagandha is important for overall health and well-being due to its adaptogenic qualities and ability to support stress resilience, energy levels, cognitive function, and immune health.

Can a Healthy Person Take Ashwagandha?

Yes, ashwagandha supplements can be taken by healthy individuals as a natural way to support overall health, stress management, and vitality. However, it's important to get advice from a healthcare professional before beginning any new supplements, especially if you have underlying health conditions or are under medications.

Best Time to Take for Better Absorption:

Ashwagandha supplements can be taken at any time of day, with or without food. However, some people prefer to take them with meals to enhance absorption. Consistency in supplementation is more important than timing.

Ashwagandha Should Combine with Which Foods for Better Absorption:

While ashwagandha supplements can be effective on their own, combining them with certain foods may enhance absorption and efficacy. Some foods that may improve the absorption of ashwagandha include:

- **Healthy fats:** Consuming ashwagandha supplements with foods rich in healthy fats, such as eggs, avocados, nuts, seeds, and extra virgin olive oil, may improve absorption due to the fat-soluble nature of some of its active compounds.
- **Black pepper:** Piperine, a compound present in black pepper, has been shown to enhance the absorption of certain nutrients and phytochemicals. Combining ashwagandha supplements with a pinch of black pepper may improve bioavailability.
- **Warm beverages:** Taking ashwagandha supplements with warm beverages like herbal tea or warm water may help relax the digestive system and enhance absorption.

Here are some common dosage recommendations for ashwagandha supplements:

- **Standardized Extracts:** Many ashwagandha supplements come in the form of standardized extracts, which contain a specific concentration of active compounds. A typical dosage range for standardized extracts is **300 mg to 600 mg** should be taken daily, split into separate doses.
- **Powder or Capsule Form:** The recommended dosage for ashwagandha powder or capsules may vary based on the concentration and potency of the specific product. It is important to follow the dosage instructions stated on the product label. If unsure, it is advisable to consult with a healthcare provider for individualized dosage recommendations.

- **Liquid Extracts or Tinctures:** Liquid extracts or tinctures of ashwagandha may have different dosing recommendations. Follow the dosage instructions given below or consult with a healthcare professional for guidance.
- **Combination Formulas:** Ashwagandha may also be found in combination formulas with other herbs or nutrients. In such cases, the recommended dosage may change depending on the particular formulation and intended use. Follow the dosage instructions given below or consult with a healthcare professional.

MELATONIN

Melatonin is a hormone chiefly generated by the pineal gland in the brain, primarily secreted in response to darkness. It plays an important role in regulating the sleep-wake cycle (circadian rhythm) and is often referred to as the **"sleep hormone."**

What is Melatonin?

Melatonin is an important hormone that governs the body's internal clock and sleep-wake cycle. It is assembled from the amino acid tryptophan, which is mainly produced in the pineal gland, a small gland situated in the brain.

Importance and Benefits of Melatonin:

- **Regulation of Sleep-Wake Cycle:** Melatonin helps synchronize the body's internal clock with the regular day-night cycle, thereby encouraging healthy sleep patterns and improving sleep quality.
- **Supports Sleep Initiation:** Melatonin levels typically rise in the evening as it gets dark, conveying to the body that it's time to sleep. Supplemental melatonin can help facilitate the onset of sleep, especially in individuals with sleep disorders or jet lag.
- **Antioxidant Properties:** Melatonin has antioxidant properties, may aid in shielding cells from oxidative damage caused by free radicals.
- **Immune Function:** Melatonin may support immune function and contribute to overall immune health.
- **Stress Reduction:** Certain research indicates that melatonin may help reduce stress and anxiety levels, particularly when used as a sleep aid to improve overall sleep quality.

Impact on Health:

Melatonin plays a crucial role in maintaining optimal sleep patterns, which are fundamental for overall health and well-being. Sufficient sleep is associated with numerous health benefits, including improved cognitive function, mood regulation, immune function, and cardiovascular health.

Evidence of Reducing Stress and Promoting Sleep:

While melatonin is primarily known for its role in promoting sleep, some research suggests that it may also have stress-reducing effects, mainly when used to improve sleep quality. However, more research is needed to fully understand the mechanisms and clinical efficacy of melatonin in reducing stress.

Can a Healthy Person Take Melatonin?

Yes, (It is not compulsory if your sleep is already good for a minimum of 6 hours.) Healthy individuals can take melatonin supplements to support overall sleep quality, regulate sleep patterns, and manage occasional sleep disturbances. However, it's important to use melatonin supplements responsibly and avoid excessive or long-term use without medical supervision.

Best Time to Take for Better Absorption:

The best time to take melatonin supplements for better absorption is typically 30 minutes to one hour before bedtime. This allows the melatonin to mimic the regular rise in melatonin levels that happens in the evening as it gets dark, helping facilitate the onset of sleep.

Melatonin for Better Absorption:

Melatonin supplements can be taken on an empty stomach or with a small snack before bedtime. While specific foods do not necessarily enhance melatonin absorption, consuming a balanced diet rich in nutrients that support sleep, such as magnesium, tryptophan, and vitamin B6, may help promote overall sleep quality.

Right Dosage:

The appropriate dosage of melatonin can vary depending on individual factors such as age, sleep patterns, and the severity of sleep disturbances. As a general guideline, starting with a low dose of **0.3 to 0.5 mg (beginning) to 1 mg** is recommended for most adults. Higher doses may be appropriate for certain individuals or under medical supervision. It's important to seek help from a healthcare professional for individual recommendations based on your needs and circumstances.

TAURINE

Taurine, an amino acid containing sulfur, is not commonly found in plant-based foods and it is not utilized for protein synthesis nor like other amino acids. Instead, it plays various important roles in the body, particularly in the brain, heart, eyes, and muscles.

What is Taurine?

Taurine is an essential amino acid that is considered conditionally essential, meaning that while the body can produce it, supplementation may be beneficial in certain circumstances. It is found in various animal-based foods and is also synthesized in small amounts in the body.

Importance and Benefits of Taurine:

- **Heart Health:** Taurine has been shown to support cardiovascular function by regulating blood pressure, reducing inflammation, and protecting against oxidative stress.
- **Brain Function:** Taurine plays a vital role in neurotransmitter regulation and may support brain function and mental health.
- **Muscle Health:** Taurine is involved in muscle contraction and helps in minimizing muscle fatigue and soreness during exercise.
- **Eye Health:** Taurine is plentiful in the retina of the eye and has the potential to safeguard against age-related macular degeneration and other eye conditions.
- **Electrolyte Balance:** Taurine helps regulate electrolyte balance in cells and may support hydration and exercise performance.

Impact on Muscle Health:

While taurine is not directly involved in muscle protein synthesis like other amino acids, it may still play a role in muscle health and exercise performance. Taurine has been shown to minimize muscle fatigue and soreness, improve exercise capacity, and enhance muscle recovery, particularly during high-intensity or prolonged exercise.

Evidence on taurine:

While taurine supplementation has been studied for its effects on exercise performance and muscle health, the evidence for its ability to directly increase muscle mass or strength is limited. However, some research suggests that taurine supplementation may improve exercise performance and reduce muscle damage and recovery, which could indirectly support muscle growth and strength gains over time, especially when combined with resistance training.

Can a Healthy Person Take Taurine?

Yes, healthy individuals can take taurine supplements to support overall health and well-being, particularly if they have specific health goals related to cardiovascular health, exercise performance, or muscle recovery. Taurine is generally considered safe when used as directed.

Best Time to Take for Better Absorption:

Taurine supplements can be taken at any time of day, with or without food. However, some people prefer to take them before or after exercise to support muscle performance and recovery. Consistency in supplementation is more important than timing.

Taurine Should Combine with Which Foods for Better Absorption:

Taurine is found in various animal-based foods, including meat, fish, poultry, and dairy products. Consuming taurine-rich foods alongside other nutrients that support muscle health, such as protein, carbohydrates, and electrolytes, may enhance absorption and effectiveness.

Right Dosage:

The appropriate dosage of taurine supplements depends upon individual factors such as age, body weight, exercise habits, and specific health goals. As a general guideline, the typical dosage of taurine supplements ranges from **500 mg to 2,000 mg per day**, taken in divided doses. It's important to seek help from a healthcare professional for individual recommendations based on your needs and circumstances.

Taurine supplementation may be beneficial for various individuals, including:

- **Athletes and Active Individuals**: Athletes and individuals engaged in regular physical activity may benefit from taurine supplementation to support exercise performance, reduce muscle fatigue, and enhance recovery. Taurine can help maintain hydration, support muscle function, and reduce oxidative stress during intense training sessions.

- **Individuals with Cardiovascular Health Concerns:** Taurine has been shown to support cardiovascular well-being through the regulation of blood pressure, reducing inflammation, and protecting against oxidative stress. Individuals with cardiovascular risk factors or conditions such as hypertension, high cholesterol, or heart disease may consider taurine supplementation as part of a comprehensive approach to heart health.

- **People with Eye Health Concerns:** Taurine is abundant in the eye's retina and plays a role in safeguarding against age-related macular degeneration and other eye conditions. Individuals at risk of eye diseases or those looking to support eye health may benefit from taurine supplementation.

- **Individuals with Neurological Conditions:** Taurine has been studied for its potential neuroprotective effects and its role in supporting cognitive function and mental health. Individuals with neurological conditions, mood disorders, or cognitive decline may consider taurine supplementation under the guidance of a healthcare professional.

- **Vegans and Vegetarians:** Taurine is primarily found in animal-based foods, and vegans and vegetarians may have lower taurine levels compared to those who consume animal products regularly. Taurine supplementation may be beneficial for individuals following vegan or vegetarian diets to ensure adequate intake of this important amino acid.

- **People Experiencing Stress or Anxiety:** Taurine has been investigated for its possible anxiolytic (anti-anxiety) properties and its ability to encourage relaxation and alleviate stress. People dealing with persistent stress, anxiety, or mood fluctuations may find taurine supplementation beneficial when incorporated into a comprehensive strategy for managing stress and enhancing emotional health.

- **Those with Liver Health Concerns:** Taurine plays a role in bile acid conjugation and liver function, and supplementation may be beneficial for individuals with liver health concerns or conditions such as non-alcoholic fatty liver disease (NAFLD) or liver damage.

Before initiating taurine supplementation, it's crucial to consult with a healthcare professional, particularly if you have any pre-existing health conditions, are pregnant or breastfeeding, or are taking medications. They can provide instruction based on your unique health situation and requirements.

BETA-ALANINE

What is Beta-Alanine?

Beta-alanine is a synthesized non-essential amino acid in the liver derived from other amino acids, particularly alanine. It is a precursor to carnosine, a dipeptide found in muscle tissue that helps buffer acidity and delay fatigue during high-intensity exercise.

Importance and Benefits of Beta-Alanine:

- **Muscle Fatigue Reduction:** Beta-alanine supplementation increases carnosine levels in muscles, which helps buffer acidity and reduce fatigue during high-intensity exercise, such as weightlifting and sprinting.
- **Exercise Performance:** Beta-alanine supplementation has been demonstrated to improve exercise performance, particularly during short-duration, high-intensity activities that rely on anaerobic metabolism.
- **Muscle Growth:** While beta-alanine does not directly stimulate muscle protein synthesis like other amino acids, its ability to enhance exercise performance and delay fatigue may indirectly support muscle growth and strength gains over a period of time, particularly when combined with resistance training.
- **Endurance Enhancement:** Beta-alanine supplementation may help increase endurance and postpone the onset of fatigue during prolonged exercise, such as endurance running or cycling.

Impact on Muscle Health:

Beta-alanine primarily impacts muscle health by increasing carnosine levels, which helps buffer acidity and delay fatigue during high-intensity exercise. By reducing muscle fatigue, beta-alanine supplementation may support exercise performance, muscle endurance, and overall muscle health.

Evidence of beta-alanine:

While beta-alanine supplementation has been shown to improve exercise performance and delay fatigue, the evidence for its direct effects on building muscle mass and strength is limited. However, some research suggests that the improvements in exercise performance and endurance resulting from beta-alanine supplementation may indirectly support muscle growth and strength gains, especially when combined with resistance training.

Only Bodybuilders Should Take Beta-Alanine?

Beta-alanine supplementation is not limited to bodybuilders and can be beneficial for individuals engaged in various forms of exercise, including athletes, recreational exercisers, and fitness enthusiasts. Anyone looking to improve exercise performance, delay fatigue, and enhance muscle endurance may consider beta-alanine supplementation, regardless of their specific fitness goals.

Best Time to Take for Better Absorption:

Beta-alanine supplements are commonly consumed in divided doses throughout the day or one time before/during a workout to maximize carnosine synthesis in muscles. The timing of beta-alanine supplementation is less critical compared to other supplements, as carnosine levels in muscles increase gradually with regular supplementation. Some individuals may experience tingling sensations (paresthesia) when taking beta-alanine, which is temporary and harmless.

Beta-alanine is often combined with other supplements that support exercise performance and muscle health, such as creatine monohydrate, branched-chain amino acids (BCAAs), and caffeine. Combining beta-alanine with creatine, in particular, may have synergistic effects on exercise performance and muscle strength.

Right Dosage:

The recommended daily intake of beta-alanine typically ranges from **4 to 6 grams**. It is recommended to start with a lower dosage and gradually increase over time to mitigate potential side effects, such as tingling sensations (paresthesia). As with any supplement, it's advisable to seek help from a healthcare professional or sports nutritionist to obtain personalized guidance based on individual requirements and circumstances.

ARGININE

Arginine, classified as a semi-essential amino acid, is produced by the body but may require supplementation in specific situations. It participates in diverse physiological functions, contributing significantly to protein synthesis, the generation of nitric oxide, and the maintenance of cardiovascular well-being.

What is Arginine?

Arginine, classified as a semi-essential amino acid, participates in a wide array of physiological functions within the body. As a precursor to nitric oxide (NO), a crucial molecule involved in vasodilation (the expansion of blood vessels), arginine has significant implications for cardiovascular well-being, exercise performance, and muscle function.

Arginine can be synthesized in the body from other amino acids, primarily citrulline. It is also obtained from dietary sources, including protein-packed foods like meat, fish, dairy products, nuts, and legumes.

Importance and Benefits of Arginine:

- **Protein Synthesis:** Arginine plays a role in protein synthesis, which is essential for muscle repair, growth, and maintenance.
- **Immune Function:** Arginine is involved in immune system regulation and may support immune function and response to infections.
- **Wound Healing:** Arginine has the ability to accelerate wound healing properties and tissue repair by increasing collagen production and enhancing blood flow to injured areas.
- **Cardiovascular Health:** Arginine supplementation may help improve endothelial function, decrease blood pressure, and mitigate the risk of cardiovascular conditions like hypertension and atherosclerosis.

Impact on Muscle Health:

Arginine may indirectly support muscle health by promoting vasodilation and increasing blood flow to muscles during exercise. Improved blood flow can enhance nutrient delivery and waste removal, potentially leading to better exercise performance, muscle recovery, and overall muscle health.

Evidence on arginine:

The evidence for arginine's direct role in building muscle and strength is limited. While arginine supplementation may improve blood flow and nutrient delivery to muscles, which could theoretically support muscle growth and recovery, the research on its effects on muscle protein synthesis and strength gains is inconclusive.

Only Bodybuilders Should Take Arginine?

Arginine supplementation is not limited to bodybuilders and can be beneficial for individuals engaged in various forms of exercise and physical activity. Anyone looking to support cardiovascular health, enhance exercise performance, promote muscle recovery, or improve overall well-being may consider arginine supplementation.

Best Time to Take Arginine for Better Absorption:

Arginine supplements are often taken before exercise or physical activity to support vasodilation and enhance blood flow to muscles (recommended). However, the timing of arginine supplementation may vary depending on individual preferences and specific goals. When consuming arginine supplements, some individuals may find that taking them on an empty stomach facilitates better absorption, while others may opt to take them alongside meals to reduce potential gastrointestinal discomfort.

Arginine Should Combine with Which Supplement for Better Absorption:

Arginine supplements may be combined with other nutrients or supplements that support exercise performance, muscle health, and overall well-being. For example, combining arginine with citrulline may enhance nitric oxide production and vasodilation, while combining arginine with branched-chain amino acids (BCAAs) may support muscle protein synthesis and recovery.

Right Dosage:

The appropriate dosage of arginine supplements changes depending on individual factors such as age, body weight, exercise habits, and specific health goals. As a general guideline, typical doses of arginine supplements range from **(0.15grams per kg, so an 80kg person should consume 80x0.15=12 grams)** or start with **6 to 8 grams** per day. It is advisable, to begin with a lower dosage and gradually increase it over time to evaluate tolerance and reduce the risk of side effects. Consulting with a healthcare provider or sports nutritionist for personalized recommendations tailored to individual needs and circumstances is recommended before starting any supplement regimen.

Who can benefit:

- **Athletes and Active Individuals**: Athletes and individuals engaged in regular physical activity may benefit from arginine supplementation to support exercise performance, improve blood flow to muscles, and enhance muscle recovery.
- **Bodybuilders and Strength Trainers**: Bodybuilders, weightlifters, and individuals engaged in resistance training may consider arginine supplementation to support muscle growth, strength gains, and workout performance.

- **Endurance Athletes:** Athletes such as runners, cyclists, and swimmers might experience performance benefits from arginine supplementation to improve blood flow, oxygen delivery, and endurance capacity during prolonged exercise.

- **Individuals with Cardiovascular Health Concerns:** Arginine supplementation may be beneficial for individuals with cardiovascular risk factors or conditions such as hypertension, atherosclerosis, or heart disease. Arginine can help improve endothelial function, lower blood pressure, and promote overall heart health.

- **Those with Poor Circulation:** Individuals experiencing poor circulation, cold extremities, or peripheral vascular disease may benefit from arginine supplementation to improve blood flow to extremities and enhance circulation.

- **People with Wound Healing Needs:** Arginine supplementation has been shown to promote wound healing properties and tissue repair by increasing collagen production, enhancing blood flow, and supporting immune function. Individuals with slow-healing wounds or surgical incisions may consider arginine supplementation under medical supervision.

- **Individuals with Erectile Dysfunction:** Arginine supplementation may help men with erectile dysfunction improve erectile function (ED) by enhancing the circulation of blood to the genital region and vascular health. However, it's important to consult with a healthcare professional before using arginine for this purpose.

- **Those Seeking Overall Health and Wellness:** Arginine supplementation may be beneficial for individuals looking to support overall health and well-being, promote immune function, and enhance nutrient delivery to cells and tissues.

CITRULLINE MALATE

What is Citrulline Malate?

Citrulline malate is a substance consisting of the amino acid citrulline combined with malic acid. It is commonly used as a dietary supplement to support exercise performance, muscle recovery, and overall health.

How It's Made:

Citrulline malate is typically produced through a chemical synthesis process that combines citrulline with malic acid to form the compound. The resulting citrulline malate powder is then used in dietary supplements.

Importance and Benefits of Citrulline Malate:

- **Increased Nitric Oxide Production:** Citrulline malate is a precursor to arginine, which is then converted into nitric oxide (NO) in the body. Nitric oxide plays a key role in widening blood vessels, promoting blood flow, and enhancing nutrient delivery to muscles during exercise.
- **Enhanced Exercise Performance:** Citrulline malate supplementation has been shown to improve exercise performance, delay fatigue, and increase endurance capacity, particularly during high-intensity or prolonged exercise.
- **Reduced Muscle Soreness:** Citrulline malate may help minimize muscle soreness and improve muscle recovery following intense exercise by promoting the clearance of metabolic waste products such as lactic acid.
- **Support for Muscle Protein Synthesis:** Citrulline malate may indirectly support muscle protein synthesis and muscle growth by enhancing exercise performance, promoting nutrient delivery to muscles, and reducing muscle fatigue during workouts.

Evidence of Building Muscle and Strength:

While citrulline malate supplementation has been shown to improve exercise performance and reduce muscle fatigue, the evidence for its direct effects on building muscle and strength is limited. However, by supporting exercise performance and recovery, citrulline malate may indirectly contribute to muscle growth and strength gains over time, especially when combined with resistance training.

Who Should Take Citrulline Malate?

Citrulline malate supplementation may be beneficial for various individuals, including athletes, bodybuilders, endurance athletes, recreational exercisers, and individuals looking to enhance exercise performance and muscle recovery and support overall health and well-being.

Best Time to Take Citrulline Malate for Better Absorption:

Citrulline malate supplements are typically taken before exercise or physical activity to support vasodilation, enhance blood flow to muscles, and improve exercise performance. Taking citrulline malate on an empty stomach may enhance absorption and effectiveness, although individual preferences and tolerance should be considered.

Supplements to Combine with for Better Absorption:

Citrulline malate may be combined with other supplements that support exercise performance, muscle health, and overall well-being. For example, combining citrulline malate with branched-chain amino acids (BCAAs), beta-alanine, or creatine monohydrate may have synergistic effects on exercise performance, muscle recovery, and muscle growth.

Right Dosage:

The appropriate dosage of citrulline malate changes depending on individual factors such as age, body weight, exercise habits, and specific health goals. As a general guideline, typical dosages of citrulline malate range from **6 to 12 grams per day, taken approximately 30 to 60 minutes before exercise**. However, it is important to consult with a healthcare professional or sports nutritionist before starting any supplement regimen. They can offer suggestions tailored to your individual needs, health status, and fitness goals. Factors like age, body weight, exercise habits, and specific health

objectives should be considered when determining the appropriate dosage

L-CARNITINE

What is L-Carnitine?

L-carnitine is a compound synthesized in the body from the amino acids lysine and methionine. It is essential for energy metabolism as it aids in the carrying of fatty acids into the mitochondria, where they undergo beta-oxidation to generate ATP (adenosine triphosphate), the body's primary energy currency.

L-Carnitine in the Human Body:

L-carnitine functions as a carrier molecule, transporting long-chain fatty acids across the inner mitochondrial membrane, enabling the metabolism for energy production. This process is essential for the oxidation of fatty acids and the production of ATP, particularly through times of increased energy demand, such as exercise.

Why It's Important to Take L-Carnitine:

While the body can synthesize L-carnitine from dietary sources and endogenous synthesis, supplementation may be beneficial in certain circumstances. L-carnitine supplementation is often used to support energy production, enhance exercise performance, promote fat metabolism, and improve overall health and well-being.

Who Should Take L-Carnitine?

L-carnitine supplementation may be beneficial for various individuals, including athletes, fitness enthusiasts, individuals looking to support fat loss, vegetarians and vegans, older adults, and individuals with certain health conditions or deficiencies. It may also be used as a therapeutic supplement under medical supervision for specific health concerns.

Impact on Fat Loss:

L-carnitine is often marketed as a fat loss supplement due to its role in breakdown of fatty acids. By transportation of fatty acids into the mitochondria for oxidation, L-carnitine may enhance fat metabolism and energy production, potentially leading to increased fat utilization during exercise and improved body composition over time.

Evidence on carnitine:

While L-carnitine supplementation may support energy metabolism and exercise performance, the evidence for its direct effects on building muscle and strength is limited. Some studies have suggested potential benefits for muscle recovery, oxidative stress reduction, and exercise capacity, but more research is needed to establish conclusive evidence.

Do Vegans Should Supplement with L-Carnitine?

Vegans and vegetarians may have lower L-carnitine levels compared to those who eat animal products on an everyday basis, as L-carnitine is primarily found in meat, fish, and dairy products. While the body can synthesize L-carnitine from dietary sources of lysine and methionine, supplementation may be considered for individuals following plant-based diets to ensure adequate intake of this important compound.

Best Time to Take L-Carnitine for Better Absorption and Fat Loss:

L-carnitine supplements are often taken before exercise or physical activity to enhance fat metabolism, energy production, and exercise performance. Consuming L-carnitine supplements with carbohydrates may enhance absorption and utilization, as insulin release stimulated by carbohydrate consumption can promote the uptake of L-carnitine into muscle cells. In case you are on a calorie-restricted diet, consume l-carnitine on an empty stomach without carbohydrates before a slow/moderate steady cardio for best fat loss results.

L-carnitine Should Combine with Which Supplement for Better Absorption:

L-carnitine supplements may be combined with other nutrients or supplements that support energy metabolism, exercise performance, and fat loss. For example, combining L-carnitine with caffeine, green tea extract, or other thermogenic compounds may have synergistic effects on fat metabolism and energy expenditure.

Right Dosage:

The suitable dosage of L-carnitine supplements may differ based on individual factors like age, weight, exercise routines, and health objectives. Generally, L-carnitine supplements are taken in doses ranging from **(500 mg to 2,000 mg per day)**, divided into multiple doses. It is recommended to start with a lower dosage and incrementally raise it to gauge tolerance and reduce the likelihood of adverse effects. Before starting any supplement regimen, it is wise to seek help from a healthcare professional or sports nutritionist for tailored guidance according to specific requirements and conditions.

GLUCOSAMINE & CHONDROITIN

What is Glucosamine & Chondroitin?

- Glucosamine is a naturally arising compound in the body, especially in cartilage. It plays a role in the development and restoration of cartilage and other connective tissues

- Chondroitin is a complex sugar molecule (glycosaminoglycan) that is also present in cartilage. It contributes to maintaining the structural strength and integrity of cartilage and other joint tissues

Physiology of Glucosamine & Chondroitin:

- Glucosamine and chondroitin are elements of the extracellular matrix of cartilage, where they play a crucial role in maintaining joint structure and function. They are involved in the synthesis and repair of cartilage tissue and help cushion and lubricate the joints.

Why It's Important to Take Glucosamine & Chondroitin:

- Glucosamine and chondroitin supplements are frequently utilized to support joint health and to reduce symptoms of osteoarthritis, a condition marked by the decline of cartilage and inflammation in the joints

Who Should Take Glucosamine & Chondroitin?

- Glucosamine and chondroitin supplements may be favorable for individuals experiencing joint pain, stiffness, or inflammation associated with osteoarthritis or other joint conditions.
- They are often used by older adults, athletes, and individuals with a history of joint injuries or wear and tear.

Impact on Joint Health:

- Glucosamine and chondroitin may help improve joint function, decrease pain, and slow the progression of osteoarthritis by supporting cartilage repair and regeneration, reducing inflammation, and promoting joint lubrication.

Evidence of Joint Strength:

- While glucosamine and chondroitin supplements have been widely used for joint health, the scientific evidence supporting their effectiveness remains mixed and inconclusive. Some studies have shown modest benefits in reducing pain and enhancing function in individuals with osteoarthritis, while others have found no significant effects.

Do Vegans Should Supplement with Glucosamine & Chondroitin?

- Glucosamine is typically derived from shellfish shells, while chondroitin is often sourced from animal cartilage, such as bovine or shark cartilage. As such, traditional glucosamine and chondroitin supplements may not be suitable for vegans. However, there are plant-based alternatives available, such as glucosamine derived from fermented corn or mushrooms.

Best Time to Take Glucosamine & Chondroitin for Better Absorption:

- Glucosamine and chondroitin supplements are commonly taken with meals to enhance absorption. Consuming them with food allows for better digestion and absorption of the active compounds.

Glucosamine & Chondroitin Should Combine with Which Supplement for Better Absorption:

- Glucosamine and chondroitin supplements may be combined with other nutrients or supplements that support joint health, such as vitamin D, omega-3 fish oil, and vitamins C and E. These nutrients may help enhance the effectiveness of glucosamine and chondroitin in promoting joint function and reducing inflammation.

Right Dosage:

- The appropriate dosage of glucosamine and chondroitin may differ based on individual factors such as age, body weight, severity of symptoms, and specific health goals. Typical dosages may range from **1,500 to 2000 milligrams of glucosamine and 800 to 1,200 milligrams of chondroitin per day**, taken in divided doses. It's important to follow the dosage recommendations on the supplement label or seek guidance from a healthcare provider for tailored recommendations based on individual needs and circumstances.

PREBIOTICS & PROBIOTICS

What are Prebiotics & Probiotics?

- Prebiotics: Prebiotics are fibers (non-digestible) that act as food source for advantageous bacteria in the gut. They help nourish and support the growth of these beneficial bacteria, supporting a healthy balance of gut microbiota.

- Probiotics: Probiotics are microorganisms that provide health benefits when ingested in sufficient quantities. They include various strains of beneficial bacteria (such as Lactobacillus and Bifidobacterium) and yeasts (such as Saccharomyces boulardii).

Function of Prebiotics & Probiotics:

- Prebiotics: Prebiotics help feed and stimulate the growth of helpful bacteria (good bacteria) in the gut, supporting a healthy balance of gut microbiota. They help improve digestion, support immune function, and decrease the risk of certain digestive disorders.

- Probiotics: Probiotics helps restore and maintain a healthy gut microbiota by developing beneficial bacteria into the digestive tract. They support digestion, enhance immune function, and may decrease symptoms of digestive disorders such as (IBS) irritable bowel syndrome, (IBS) inflammatory bowel disease, and diarrhea.

Why It's Important to Take Prebiotics & Probiotics:

- Prebiotics and probiotics play complementary roles in promoting gut health. They promote a healthy balance of gut microbiota, which is important for digestion, nutrient absorption, immune function, and overall well-being.

- Factors such as poor diet, antibiotics, stress and certain medical conditions can disturb the balance of gut microbiota, which leads to digestive problems and other health issues. Supplementing with prebiotics and probiotics may help restore and support gut health in these situations.

Who Should Take Prebiotics & Probiotics:

- Prebiotics and probiotics may be beneficial for individuals experiencing digestive problems, such as bloating, gas, constipation, diarrhea, or symptoms of digestive disorders like IBS or IBD.
- They may also be recommended for individuals looking to support overall gut health, enhance immune function, or maintain digestive balance during or after antibiotic treatment.

Evidence of Gut Health Benefits:

- There is growing evidence supporting the benefits of prebiotics and probiotics for gut health. Clinical studies have shown that supplementation with prebiotics and probiotics can help reduce symptoms of digestive disorders, improve bowel regularity, support immune function, and decrease the risk of antibiotic-associated diarrhea and other gastrointestinal issues.

Do Vegans Should Supplement with Prebiotics & Probiotics?

- Prebiotics and probiotics are naturally found in a lot of plant-based foods, like vegetables, fruits, whole grains, legumes, and fermented foods. However, individuals following a vegan diet may have lower intakes of certain prebiotics and probiotics found in animal-based foods. In such cases, supplementation with vegan-friendly prebiotic and probiotic supplements may be beneficial to ensure adequate intake and support gut health.

Best Time to Take Prebiotics & Probiotics Supplements for Better Absorption:

- Prebiotics and probiotics can be taken at any time of day, with or without food. However, some people find it beneficial to take them with meals to minimize potential gastrointestinal discomfort and improve absorption. Taking them consistently at the same time each day may also help maintain a healthy balance of gut microbiota.

Prebiotics & Probiotics Should Combine with Which Food for Better Absorption:

- Prebiotics and probiotics can be consumed as supplements or obtained from dietary sources. Foods rich in prebiotics include **garlic, onions, leeks, asparagus, green bananas, and whole grains. Fermented foods such as yogurt, kombucha, fermented rice, idli, sauerkraut, kimchi, and miso are good sources of probiotics.**

Right Dosage:

- The appropriate dosage of prebiotics and probiotics can alter depending on individual factors such as age, health status, and specific health goals. Dosages of prebiotic and probiotic supplements are typically measured in colony-forming units (CFUs) for probiotics and grams for prebiotics. It's important to follow the dosage recommendations on the supplement label or seek guidance from a healthcare provider for tailored recommendations based on individual needs and circumstances.

COLLAGEN

What is Collagen?

- Collagen is a robust and resilient protein that gives strength, structure, and support to various tissues in the body, including skin, bones, muscles, tendons, ligaments, and cartilage. It is a combination of amino acids, primarily glycine, proline, and hydroxyproline, and forms long, fibrous chains that give tissues their elasticity and resilience.

Function of Collagen in the Human Body:

- Collagen serves several important functions in the body, including:
    - Providing structural support and strength to tissues and organs
    - Maintaining the integrity and elasticity of the skin, promoting a youthful appearance
    - Supporting bone health and density, contributing to bone strength and flexibility
    - Enhancing joint function and mobility by providing cushioning and lubrication to joints
    - Supporting muscle and tendon health by providing structural support and promoting tissue repair

Why It's Important to Take Collagen:

- Collagen production declines naturally with age, leading to changes in skin elasticity, joint stiffness, and bone density. Supplementing with collagen may help support and maintain the health and integrity of these tissues, enhancing overall health and well-being.

Different Types of Collagen:

- There are multiple types of collagen found in the human body, each with specific functions and distribution:
  - **Type I:** Found in skin, bones, tendons, ligaments, and teeth; provides structural support and strength.
  - **Type II:** Found in cartilage, particularly in joints; provides cushioning and shock absorption.
  - **Type III:** Found in skin, blood vessels, and internal organs; contributes to skin elasticity and vascular health.
  - **Type IV:** Found in basement membranes; provides structural support and filtration.
  - **Type V:** Found in cell surfaces and hair; plays an important role in tissue development and organization.

Functions of Different Types of Collagen:

- Each type of collagen has unique functions and distribution in the body, contributing to the structure, strength, and function of specific tissues and organs.

Does Supplementing with Collagen Have Strong Evidence?

- While there is growing evidence supporting the benefits of collagen supplementation for skin health, joint function, and bone density, more research is needed to establish conclusive evidence of its effectiveness. Some studies have shown positive effects of collagen supplementation on skin elasticity, hydration, and wrinkle reduction, as well as improvements in joint pain and mobility.

Do Vegans Should Supplement with Collagen?

- Traditional collagen supplements are obtained from animal sources, such as **bovine (cow)** or **marine (fish) collagen.** However, there are vegan-friendly alternatives available, such as collagen peptides derived from plant sources like algae or bacteria. Vegans and vegetarians may consider supplementing with these plant-based collagen alternatives to support their collagen needs.

Best Form of Collagen:

- Collagen supplements are available in various forms, including collagen peptides, hydrolyzed collagen, collagen powders, collagen capsules, and collagen drinks. **Collagen peptides, marine collagen, and hydrolyzed collagen** are broken down into smaller, more easily absorbed molecules, making them a popular choice for supplementation.

Collagen Should Combine with Which Food for Better Absorption:

- Collagen supplements can be taken on an empty stomach or with meals. Consuming collagen with vitamin C-rich foods or supplements may enhance absorption, as vitamin C is necessary for collagen synthesis in the body.

Right Dosage:

- The suitable amount of collagen supplements can vary with factors like age, overall health, and specific health objectives. Standard doses of collagen peptides or hydrolyzed collagen typically fall between **5 to 15 grams** daily, administered in separate doses. Adhering to the dosage instructions on the supplement packaging or seeking advice from a healthcare provider for tailored recommendations according to individual requirements and conditions is crucial.

GLYCINE

Glycine is a non-essential amino acid that plays multiple roles in the human body. It is a fundamental component in the construction of protein and participates in numerous metabolic processes. It's also involved in the synthesis of important molecules such as glutathione, creatine, and collagen.

How It's Made:

Glycine can be synthesized in the body from other amino acids, primarily serine. It's also obtained from dietary sources such as protein-rich foods like meat, fish, dairy products, legumes, and certain grains.

Effect on Sleep Health:

- Research has explored the potential impacts of glycine on various aspects of sleep quality and relaxation. Research suggests that glycine supplementation may promote sleep quality by:
    - Reduce the duration of time needed to initiate sleep (sleep onset latency)
    - Improving sleep efficiency.
    - Enhancing subjective measures of sleep quality.
- Glycine might exert a soothing influence on the nervous system, promoting relaxation and diminishing anxiety, potentially enhancing sleep quality.

Dosage:

- The effective dosage of glycine for improving sleep quality can vary among individuals.
- Clinical studies have used doses ranging from **3 grams to 5 grams** taken before bedtime.
- Optimal effects may be achieved with varying dosage levels, as some individuals may find lower doses sufficient, while others may necessitate higher amounts to attain the desired benefits.

Who Should Take Glycine?

- Individuals experiencing sleep disturbances or insomnia may benefit from glycine supplementation to improve sleep quality and promote relaxation.
- People are looking for natural approaches to support overall sleep health and relaxation without the side effects associated with some sleep medications.

Health Benefits and Gut Health:

- **Joint Health:** Glycine is a component of collagen, the predominant structural protein found in connective tissues like bones, joints, and skin. Supplementing with glycine may promote joint health and may help reduce symptoms of conditions like osteoarthritis.
- **Gut Health:** Glycine participates in the production of glutathione, an antioxidant that contributes to the regulation of protecting the gut lining and supporting overall gut health. Additionally, glycine may have anti-inflammatory effects that can benefit gut health.

Timing for Better Absorption:

- Glycine supplements can be taken before bedtime to support relaxation and promote better sleep quality.
- Some individuals may also benefit from dividing their glycine dosage throughout the day, such as taking smaller doses in the evening and before bedtime

PLANNER

A NEW BEGINNING

Welcome!

BODY MEASUREMENTS CHART

Date: _______________________

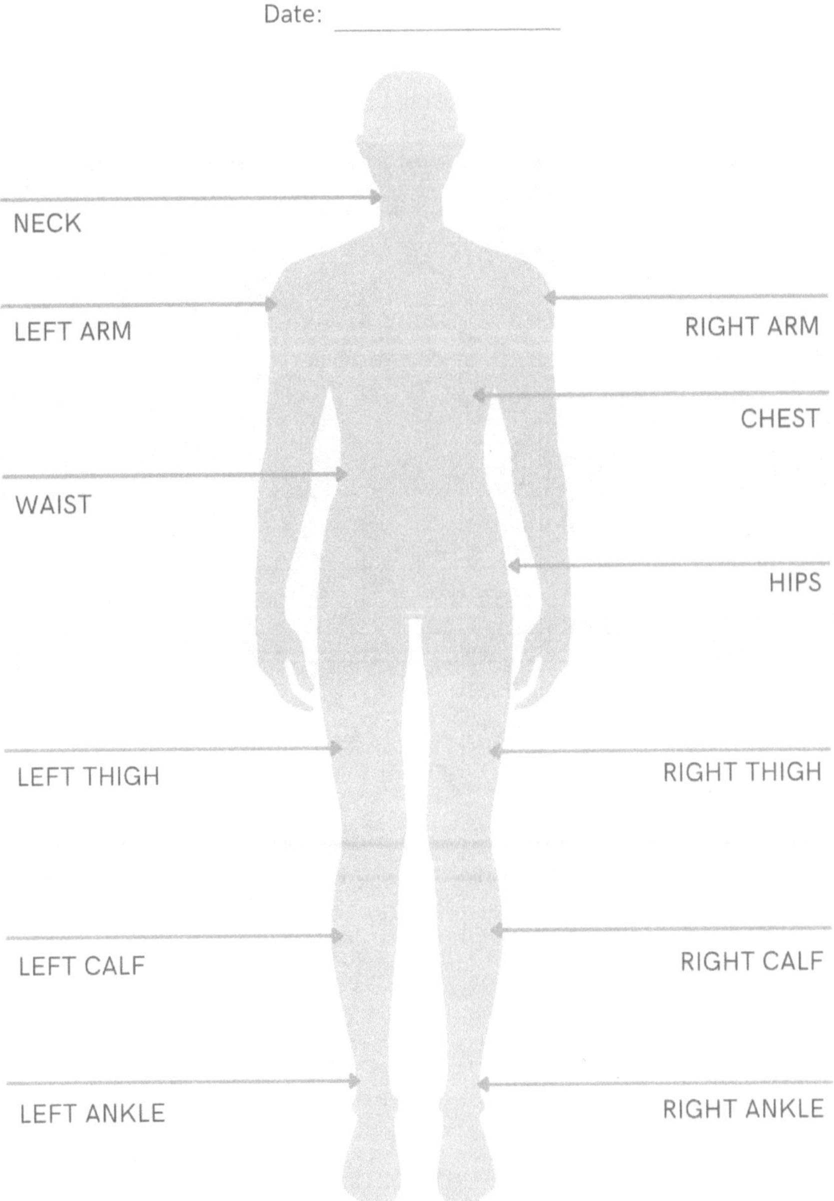

Muscle Mastery 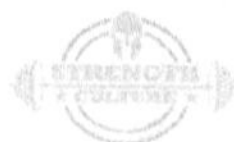

DATE: __________

M   T   W   T   F   S   S

DAILY STEPS: __________   **MUSCLE GROUP :** __________

DAILY GOALS : __________   **TOTAL TIME:** __________

EXERCISE LOG

	EXERCISE	Sets	Reps	Intensity	1ST SET	2ND SET	3RD SET	4TH SET	5TH SET	REST
1										
2										
3										
4										
5										
6										
7										
8										
9										
10										

MOOD AND ENERGY LEVELS

CARDIO

TYPE	TIME	CALORIES BURNED'

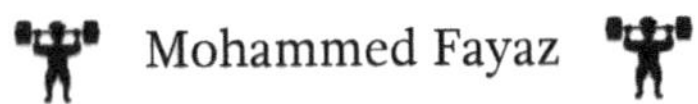

NUTRITION TRACKER

BODY WEIGHT: _______________________________

BODY FAT %: _______________________________

SLEEP (HOURS): _______________________________

SUPPLEMENTS: _______________________________

Water

FOOD/MEAL	SERV	CARBS	PROTEIN	FAT	CALS
CALORIES CONSUMED					

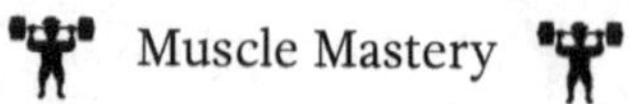

Muscle Mastery

DATE: [ ]

M   T   W   T   F   S   S

DAILY STEPS: _______________   **MUSCLE GROUP :** _______________

DAILY GOALS : _______________   **TOTAL TIME:** _______________

EXERCISE LOG

	EXERCISE	Sets	Reps	Intensity	1ST SET	2ND SET	3RD SET	4TH SET	5TH SET	REST
1										
2										
3										
4										
5										
6										
7										
8										
9										
10										

MOOD AND ENERGY LEVELS

CARDIO

TYPE	TIME	CALORIES BURNED'

NUTRITION TRACKER

BODY WEIGHT: _______________________

BODY FAT %: _______________________

SLEEP (HOURS): _______________________

SUPPLEMENTS: _______________________

Water

FOOD/MEAL	SERV	CARBS	PROTEIN	FAT	CALS
CALORIES CONSUMED					

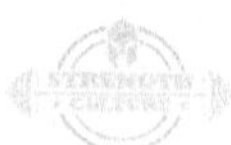 Muscle Mastery

DATE:

M T W T F S S

DAILY STEPS:

MUSCLE GROUP :

DAILY GOALS :

TOTAL TIME:

EXERCISE LOG

	EXERCISE	Sets	Reps	Intensity	1ST SET	2ND SET	3RD SET	4TH SET	5TH SET	REST
1										
2										
3										
4										
5										
6										
7										
8										
9										
10										

MOOD AND ENERGY LEVELS

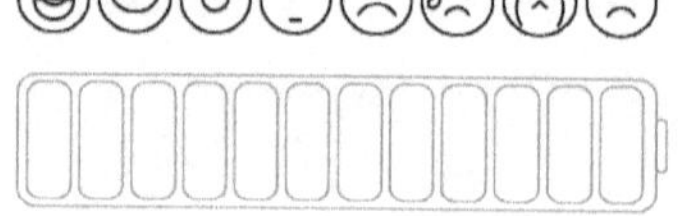

CARDIO

TYPE	TIME	CALORIES BURNED'

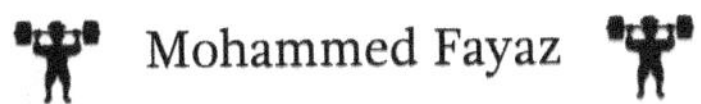

NUTRITION TRACKER

BODY WEIGHT: ______________________

BODY FAT %: ______________________

SLEEP (HOURS): ______________________

SUPPLEMENTS: ______________________

Water

FOOD/MEAL	SERV	CARBS	PROTEIN	FAT	CALS
CALORIES CONSUMED					

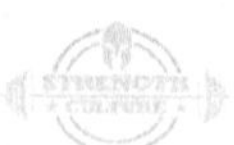

Muscle Mastery

DATE: [　　　　　　　　]

M　T　W　T　F　S　S

DAILY STEPS:

MUSCLE GROUP:

DAILY GOALS:

TOTAL TIME:

EXERCISE LOG

	EXERCISE	Sets	Reps	Intensity	1ST SET	2ND SET	3RD SET	4TH SET	5TH SET	REST
1										
2										
3										
4										
5										
6										
7										
8										
9										
10										

MOOD AND ENERGY LEVELS

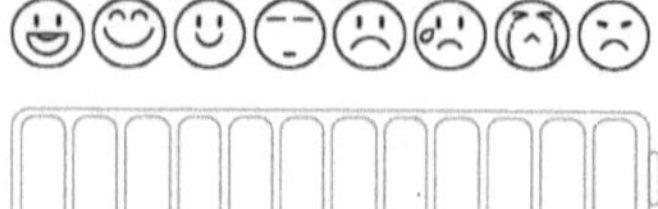

CARDIO

TYPE	TIME	CALORIES BURNED'

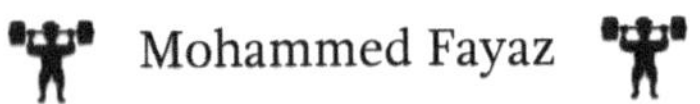 Mohammed Fayaz

NUTRITION TRACKER

BODY WEIGHT: _______________________

BODY FAT %: _______________________

SLEEP (HOURS): _______________________

SUPPLEMENTS: _______________________

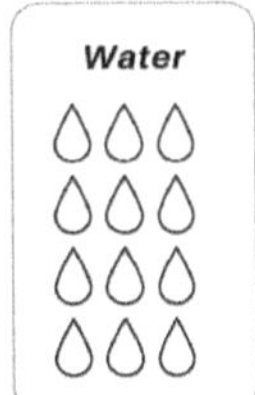

FOOD/MEAL	SERV	CARBS	PROTEIN	FAT	CALS
CALORIES CONSUMED					

Muscle Mastery 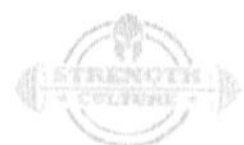

DATE:

M   T   W   T   F   S   S

DAILY STEPS: **MUSCLE GROUP :**

DAILY GOALS :   **TOTAL TIME:**

EXERCISE LOG

	EXERCISE	Sets	Reps	Intensity	1ST SET	2ND SET	3RD SET	4TH SET	5TH SET	REST
1										
2										
3										
4										
5										
6										
7										
8										
9										
10										

MOOD AND ENERGY LEVELS

CARDIO

TYPE	TIME	CALORIES BURNED'

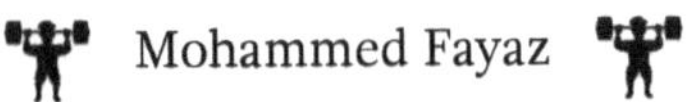

NUTRITION TRACKER

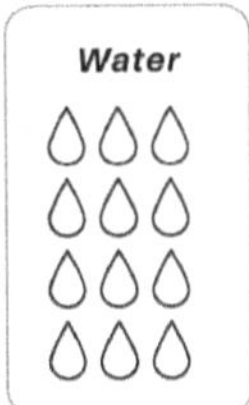

BODY WEIGHT: _______________________________

BODY FAT %: _______________________________

SLEEP (HOURS): _______________________________

SUPPLEMENTS: _______________________________

FOOD/MEAL	SERV	CARBS	PROTEIN	FAT	CALS
CALORIES CONSUMED					

Muscle Mastery

DATE:

M   T   W   T   F   S   S

DAILY STEPS:

MUSCLE GROUP :

DAILY GOALS :

TOTAL TIME:

EXERCISE LOG

	EXERCISE	Sets	Reps	Intensity	1ST SET	2ND SET	3RD SET	4TH SET	5TH SET	REST
1										
2										
3										
4										
5										
6										
7										
8										
9										
10										

MOOD AND ENERGY LEVELS

CARDIO

TYPE	TIME	CALORIES BURNED'

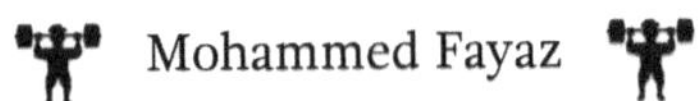

NUTRITION TRACKER

BODY WEIGHT: ____________________

BODY FAT %: ____________________

SLEEP (HOURS): ____________________

SUPPLEMENTS: ____________________

Water

FOOD/MEAL	SERV	CARBS	PROTEIN	FAT	CALS
CALORIES CONSUMED					

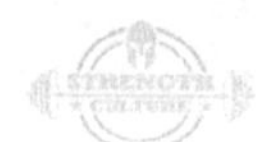

Muscle Mastery

DATE:

M   T   W   T   F   S   S

DAILY STEPS: **MUSCLE GROUP :**

DAILY GOALS :   **TOTAL TIME:**

EXERCISE LOG

	EXERCISE	Sets	Reps	Intensity	1ST SET	2ND SET	3RD SET	4TH SET	5TH SET	REST
1										
2										
3										
4										
5										
6										
7										
8										
9										
10										

MOOD AND ENERGY LEVELS

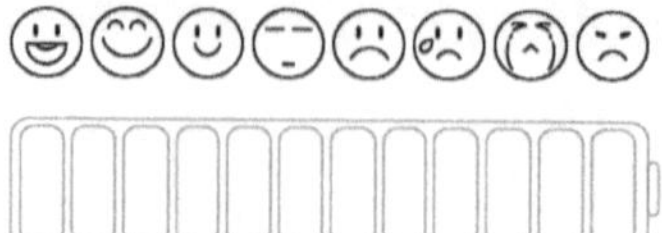

CARDIO

TYPE	TIME	CALORIES BURNED'

NUTRITION TRACKER

BODY WEIGHT: __________________________

BODY FAT %: __________________________

SLEEP (HOURS): ________________________

SUPPLEMENTS: __________________________

Water

FOOD/MEAL	SERV	CARBS	PROTEIN	FAT	CALS
CALORIES CONSUMED					

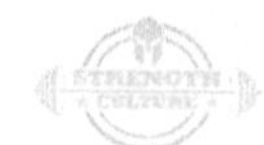

Muscle Mastery

DATE: __________________

M   T   W   T   F   S   S

DAILY STEPS: __________________

MUSCLE GROUP : __________________

DAILY GOALS : __________________

TOTAL TIME: __________________

EXERCISE LOG

	EXERCISE	Sets	Reps	Intensity	1ST SET	2ND SET	3RD SET	4TH SET	5TH SET	REST
1										
2										
3										
4										
5										
6										
7										
8										
9										
10										

MOOD AND ENERGY LEVELS

CARDIO

TYPE	TIME	CALORIES BURNED'

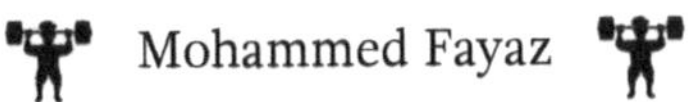

NUTRITION TRACKER

BODY WEIGHT: _______________________________

BODY FAT %: _______________________________

SLEEP (HOURS): _______________________________

SUPPLEMENTS: _______________________________

Water

FOOD/MEAL	SERV	CARBS	PROTEIN	FAT	CALS
CALORIES CONSUMED					

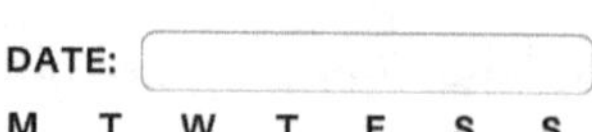 # Muscle Mastery 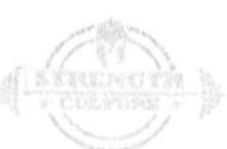

DATE: [ ]

M T W T F S S

DAILY STEPS:

MUSCLE GROUP :

DAILY GOALS :

TOTAL TIME:

EXERCISE LOG

	EXERCISE	Sets	Reps	Intensity	1ST SET	2ND SET	3RD SET	4TH SET	5TH SET	REST
1										
2										
3										
4										
5										
6										
7										
8										
9										
10										

MOOD AND ENERGY LEVELS

CARDIO

TYPE	TIME	CALORIES BURNED'

NUTRITION TRACKER

BODY WEIGHT: _______________________________

BODY FAT %: _______________________________

SLEEP (HOURS): _______________________________

SUPPLEMENTS: _______________________________

Water

FOOD/MEAL	SERV	CARBS	PROTEIN	FAT	CALS
CALORIES CONSUMED					

Muscle Mastery 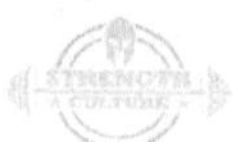

DATE: [ ]

M   T   W   T   F   S   S

DAILY STEPS: ___________________

MUSCLE GROUP: ___________________

DAILY GOALS: ___________________

TOTAL TIME: ___________________

EXERCISE LOG

	EXERCISE	Sets	Reps	Intensity	1ST SET	2ND SET	3RD SET	4TH SET	5TH SET	REST
1										
2										
3										
4										
5										
6										
7										
8										
9										
10										

MOOD AND ENERGY LEVELS

CARDIO

TYPE	TIME	CALORIES BURNED'

NUTRITION TRACKER

BODY WEIGHT: ___________________________

BODY FAT %: ___________________________

SLEEP (HOURS): ___________________________

SUPPLEMENTS: ___________________________

Water

FOOD/MEAL	SERV	CARBS	PROTEIN	FAT	CALS
CALORIES CONSUMED					

Muscle Mastery 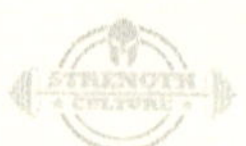

DATE: ____________

M   T   W   T   F   S   S

DAILY STEPS: ____________ **MUSCLE GROUP:** ____________

DAILY GOALS: ____________ **TOTAL TIME:** ____________

EXERCISE LOG

	EXERCISE	Sets	Reps	Intensity	1ST SET	2ND SET	3RD SET	4TH SET	5TH SET	REST
1										
2										
3										
4										
5										
6										
7										
8										
9										
10										

MOOD AND ENERGY LEVELS

CARDIO

TYPE	TIME	CALORIES BURNED'

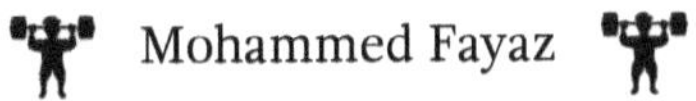

NUTRITION TRACKER

BODY WEIGHT: _______________________

BODY FAT %: _______________________

SLEEP (HOURS): _______________________

SUPPLEMENTS: _______________________

Water

FOOD/MEAL	SERV	CARBS	PROTEIN	FAT	CALS
CALORIES CONSUMED					

Muscle Mastery

DATE: ____________

M   T   W   T   F   S   S

DAILY STEPS: ______________   **MUSCLE GROUP :** ______________

DAILY GOALS : ______________   **TOTAL TIME:** ______________

EXERCISE LOG

	EXERCISE	Sets	Reps	Intensity	1ST SET	2ND SET	3RD SET	4TH SET	5TH SET	REST
1										
2										
3										
4										
5										
6										
7										
8										
9										
10										

MOOD AND ENERGY LEVELS

CARDIO

TYPE	TIME	CALORIES BURNED'

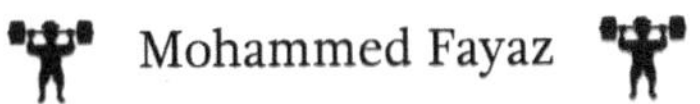

NUTRITION TRACKER

BODY WEIGHT: _______________________________

BODY FAT %: _______________________________

SLEEP (HOURS): _______________________________

SUPPLEMENTS: _______________________________

Water

FOOD/MEAL	SERV	CARBS	PROTEIN	FAT	CALS
CALORIES CONSUMED					

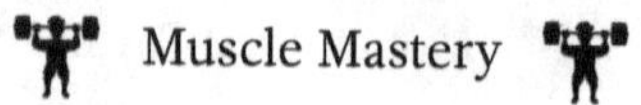 Muscle Mastery 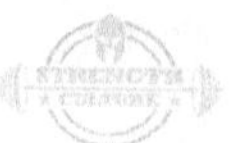

DATE:

M   T   W   T   F   S   S

DAILY STEPS:

MUSCLE GROUP:

DAILY GOALS:

TOTAL TIME:

EXERCISE LOG

	EXERCISE	Sets	Reps	Intensity	1ST SET	2ND SET	3RD SET	4TH SET	5TH SET	REST
1										
2										
3										
4										
5										
6										
7										
8										
9										
10										

MOOD AND ENERGY LEVELS

CARDIO

TYPE	TIME	CALORIES BURNED'

NUTRITION TRACKER

BODY WEIGHT: _______________________

BODY FAT %: _______________________

SLEEP (HOURS): _______________________

SUPPLEMENTS: _______________________

Water

FOOD/MEAL	SERV	CARBS	PROTEIN	FAT	CALS
CALORIES CONSUMED					

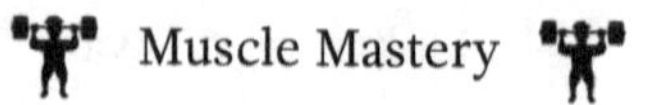

Muscle Mastery

DATE: ________________

M   T   W   T   F   S   S

DAILY STEPS: ____________________

MUSCLE GROUP : ____________________

DAILY GOALS : ____________________

TOTAL TIME: ____________________

EXERCISE LOG

	EXERCISE	Sets	Reps	Intensity	1ST SET	2ND SET	3RD SET	4TH SET	5TH SET	REST
1										
2										
3										
4										
5										
6										
7										
8										
9										
10										

MOOD AND ENERGY LEVELS

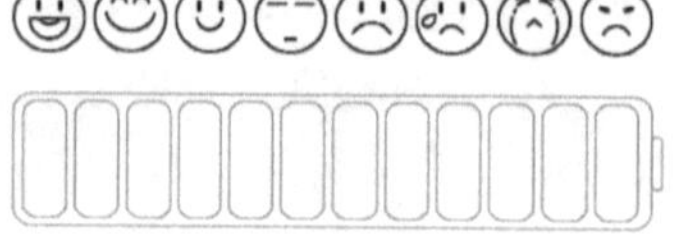

CARDIO

TYPE	TIME	CALORIES BURNED'

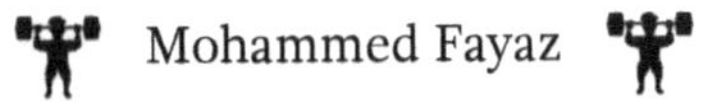

NUTRITION TRACKER

BODY WEIGHT: ___________________________

BODY FAT %: ___________________________

SLEEP (HOURS): ___________________________

SUPPLEMENTS: ___________________________

Water

FOOD/MEAL	SERV	CARBS	PROTEIN	FAT	CALS
CALORIES CONSUMED					

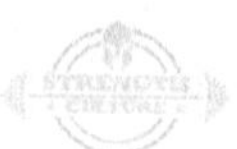

Muscle Mastery

DATE: __________

M T W T F S S

DAILY STEPS:

MUSCLE GROUP : __________

DAILY GOALS : __________

TOTAL TIME: __________

EXERCISE LOG

	EXERCISE	Sets	Reps	Intensity	1ST SET	2ND SET	3RD SET	4TH SET	5TH SET	REST
1										
2										
3										
4										
5										
6										
7										
8										
9										
10										

MOOD AND ENERGY LEVELS

CARDIO

TYPE	TIME	CALORIES BURNED'

NUTRITION TRACKER

BODY WEIGHT: ___________________________

BODY FAT %: ___________________________

SLEEP (HOURS): ___________________________

SUPPLEMENTS: ___________________________

Water

FOOD/MEAL	SERV	CARBS	PROTEIN	FAT	CALS
CALORIES CONSUMED					

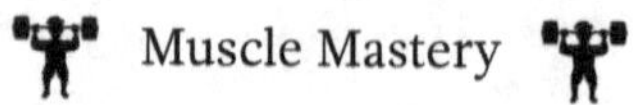

Muscle Mastery

DATE:

M   T   W   T   F   S   S

DAILY STEPS:

MUSCLE GROUP :

DAILY GOALS :

TOTAL TIME:

EXERCISE LOG

	EXERCISE	Sets	Reps	Intensity	1ST SET	2ND SET	3RD SET	4TH SET	5TH SET	REST
1										
2										
3										
4										
5										
6										
7										
8										
9										
10										

MOOD AND ENERGY LEVELS

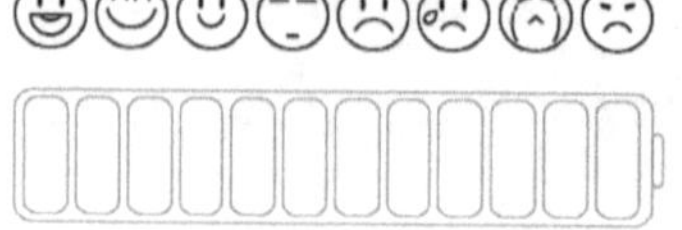

CARDIO

TYPE	TIME	CALORIES BURNED'

NUTRITION TRACKER

BODY WEIGHT: _______________________________

BODY FAT %: _______________________________

SLEEP (HOURS): _______________________________

SUPPLEMENTS: _______________________________

Water

FOOD/MEAL	SERV	CARBS	PROTEIN	FAT	CALS
CALORIES CONSUMED					

Muscle Mastery 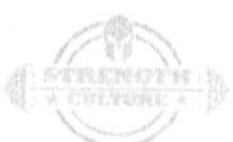

DATE: ____________

M   T   W   T   F   S   S

DAILY STEPS: ____________

MUSCLE GROUP : ____________

DAILY GOALS : ____________

TOTAL TIME: ____________

EXERCISE LOG

	EXERCISE	Sets	Reps	Intensity	1ST SET	2ND SET	3RD SET	4TH SET	5TH SET	REST
1										
2										
3										
4										
5										
6										
7										
8										
9										
10										

MOOD AND ENERGY LEVELS

CARDIO

TYPE	TIME	CALORIES BURNED'

NUTRITION TRACKER

BODY WEIGHT: _______________________________

BODY FAT %: _______________________________

SLEEP (HOURS): _______________________________

SUPPLEMENTS: _______________________________

Water

FOOD/MEAL	SERV	CARBS	PROTEIN	FAT	CALS
CALORIES CONSUMED					

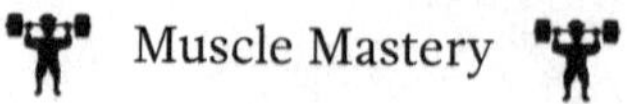 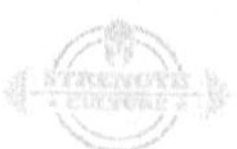

Muscle Mastery

DATE: __________
M   T   W   T   F   S   S

DAILY STEPS: __________   **MUSCLE GROUP :** __________

DAILY GOALS : __________   **TOTAL TIME:** __________

EXERCISE LOG

	EXERCISE	Sets	Reps	Intensity	1ST SET	2ND SET	3RD SET	4TH SET	5TH SET	REST
1										
2										
3										
4										
5										
6										
7										
8										
9										
10										

MOOD AND ENERGY LEVELS

CARDIO

TYPE	TIME	CALORIES BURNED'

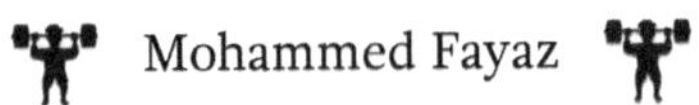

NUTRITION TRACKER

BODY WEIGHT: _______________________

BODY FAT %: _______________________

SLEEP (HOURS): _______________________

SUPPLEMENTS: _______________________

Water

FOOD/MEAL	SERV	CARBS	PROTEIN	FAT	CALS
CALORIES CONSUMED					

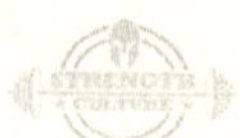

Muscle Mastery

DATE:

M   T   W   T   F   S   S

DAILY STEPS:

DAILY GOALS :

MUSCLE GROUP :

TOTAL TIME:

EXERCISE LOG

	EXERCISE	Sets	Reps	Intensity	1ST SET	2ND SET	3RD SET	4TH SET	5TH SET	REST
1										
2										
3										
4										
5										
6										
7										
8										
9										
10										

MOOD AND ENERGY LEVELS

CARDIO

TYPE	TIME	CALORIES BURNED'

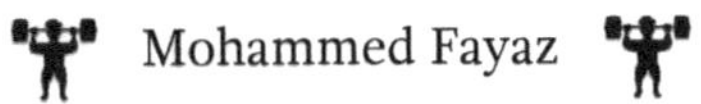 Mohammed Fayaz

NUTRITION TRACKER

BODY WEIGHT: _______________________

BODY FAT %: _______________________

SLEEP (HOURS): _______________________

SUPPLEMENTS: _______________________

Water

FOOD/MEAL	SERV	CARBS	PROTEIN	FAT	CALS
CALORIES CONSUMED					

Muscle Mastery 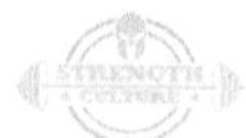

DATE:

M   T   W   T   F   S   S

DAILY STEPS:

MUSCLE GROUP:

DAILY GOALS:

TOTAL TIME:

EXERCISE LOG

	EXERCISE	Sets	Reps	Intensity	1ST SET	2ND SET	3RD SET	4TH SET	5TH SET	REST
1										
2										
3										
4										
5										
6										
7										
8										
9										
10										

MOOD AND ENERGY LEVELS

CARDIO

TYPE	TIME	CALORIES BURNED'

NUTRITION TRACKER

BODY WEIGHT: ___________________________

BODY FAT %: ___________________________

SLEEP (HOURS): ___________________________

SUPPLEMENTS: ___________________________

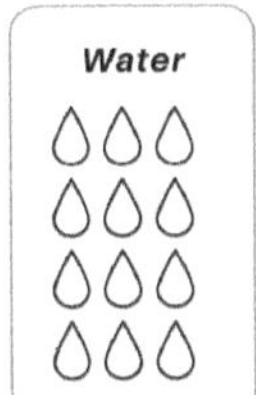

FOOD/MEAL	SERV	CARBS	PROTEIN	FAT	CALS
CALORIES CONSUMED					

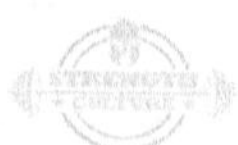

Muscle Mastery

DATE: [ ]

M T W T F S S

DAILY STEPS:

MUSCLE GROUP :

DAILY GOALS :

TOTAL TIME:

EXERCISE LOG

	EXERCISE	Sets	Reps	Intensity	1ST SET	2ND SET	3RD SET	4TH SET	5TH SET	REST
1										
2										
3										
4										
5										
6										
7										
8										
9										
10										

MOOD AND ENERGY LEVELS

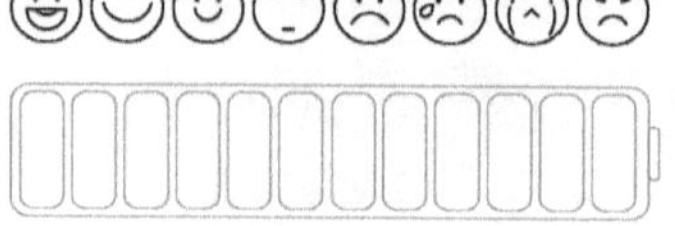

CARDIO

TYPE	TIME	CALORIES BURNED'

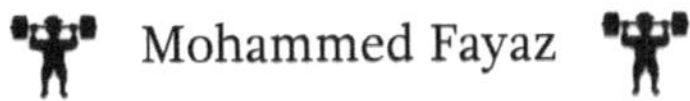

NUTRITION TRACKER

BODY WEIGHT: _______________________

BODY FAT %: _______________________

SLEEP (HOURS): _______________________

SUPPLEMENTS: _______________________

Water

FOOD/MEAL	SERV	CARBS	PROTEIN	FAT	CALS
CALORIES CONSUMED					

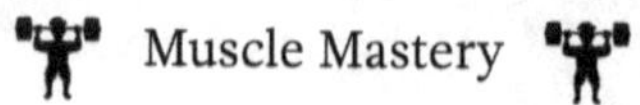

Muscle Mastery

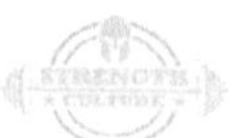

DATE: [　　　　　　　]

M　T　W　T　F　S　S

DAILY STEPS: ___________________

MUSCLE GROUP: ___________________

DAILY GOALS: ___________________

TOTAL TIME: ___________________

EXERCISE LOG

	EXERCISE	Sets	Reps	Intensity	1ST SET	2ND SET	3RD SET	4TH SET	5TH SET	REST
1										
2										
3										
4										
5										
6										
7										
8										
9										
10										

MOOD AND ENERGY LEVELS

CARDIO

TYPE	TIME	CALORIES BURNED'

NUTRITION TRACKER

BODY WEIGHT: ______________________

BODY FAT %: ______________________

SLEEP (HOURS): ______________________

SUPPLEMENTS: ______________________

Water

FOOD/MEAL	SERV	CARBS	PROTEIN	FAT	CALS
CALORIES CONSUMED					

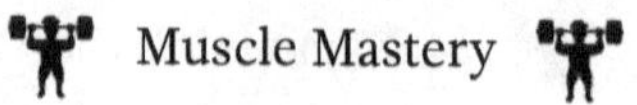

Muscle Mastery

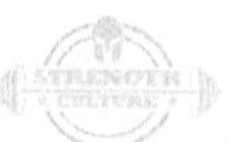

DATE:

M T W T F S S

DAILY STEPS:

MUSCLE GROUP :

DAILY GOALS :

TOTAL TIME:

EXERCISE LOG

	EXERCISE	Sets	Reps	Intensity	1ST SET	2ND SET	3RD SET	4TH SET	5TH SET	REST
1										
2										
3										
4										
5										
6										
7										
8										
9										
10										

MOOD AND ENERGY LEVELS

CARDIO

TYPE	TIME	CALORIES BURNED'

NUTRITION TRACKER

BODY WEIGHT: _______________________________

BODY FAT %: _______________________________

SLEEP (HOURS): _______________________________

SUPPLEMENTS: _______________________________

Water

FOOD/MEAL	SERV	CARBS	PROTEIN	FAT	CALS
CALORIES CONSUMED					

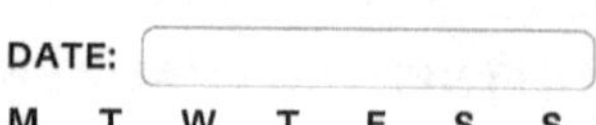 **Muscle Mastery** 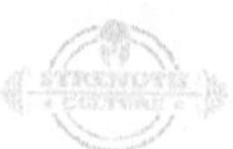

DATE:

M T W T F S S

DAILY STEPS:

MUSCLE GROUP :

DAILY GOALS :

TOTAL TIME:

EXERCISE LOG

	EXERCISE	Sets	Reps	Intensity	1ST SET	2ND SET	3RD SET	4TH SET	5TH SET	REST
1										
2										
3										
4										
5										
6										
7										
8										
9										
10										

MOOD AND ENERGY LEVELS

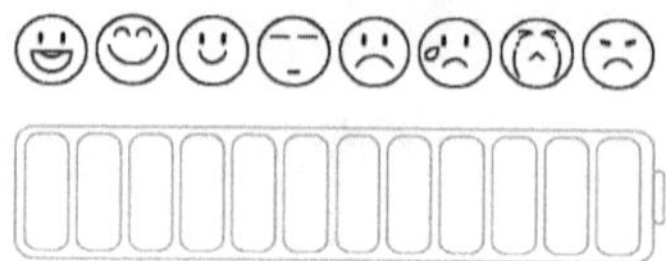

CARDIO

TYPE	TIME	CALORIES BURNED'

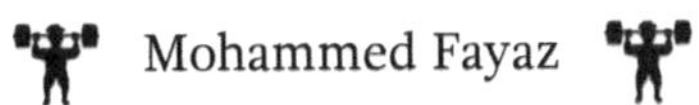

NUTRITION TRACKER

BODY WEIGHT: ______________________

BODY FAT %: ______________________

SLEEP (HOURS): ______________________

SUPPLEMENTS: ______________________

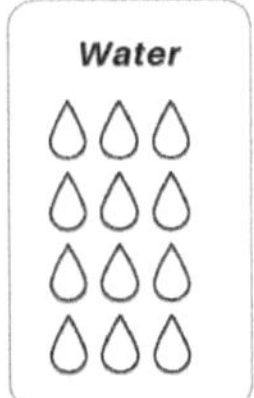

FOOD/MEAL	SERV	CARBS	PROTEIN	FAT	CALS
CALORIES CONSUMED					

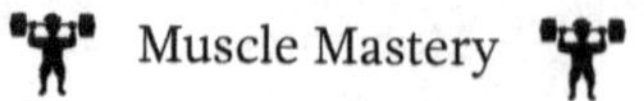 Muscle Mastery

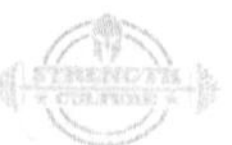

DATE: ____________________

M   T   W   T   F   S   S

DAILY STEPS: ______________________

MUSCLE GROUP : ______________________

DAILY GOALS : ______________________

TOTAL TIME: ______________________

EXERCISE LOG

	EXERCISE	Sets	Reps	Intensity	1ST SET	2ND SET	3RD SET	4TH SET	5TH SET	REST
1										
2										
3										
4										
5										
6										
7										
8										
9										
10										

MOOD AND ENERGY LEVELS

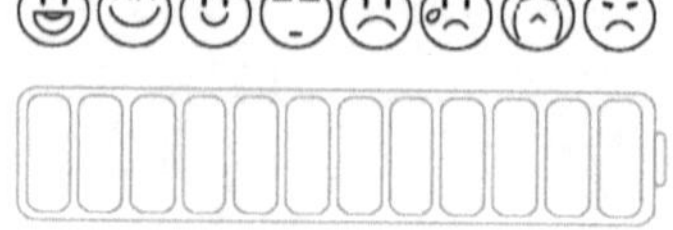

CARDIO

TYPE	TIME	CALORIES BURNED'

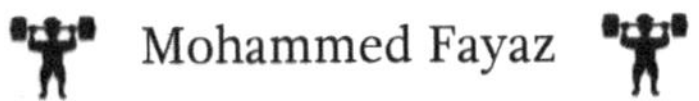

NUTRITION TRACKER

BODY WEIGHT: ______________________

BODY FAT %: ______________________

SLEEP (HOURS): ______________________

SUPPLEMENTS: ______________________

Water

FOOD/MEAL	SERV	CARBS	PROTEIN	FAT	CALS
CALORIES CONSUMED					

Muscle Mastery 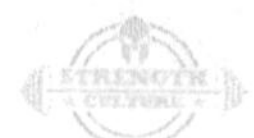

DATE: [   ]

M T W T F S S

DAILY STEPS:

MUSCLE GROUP:

DAILY GOALS:

TOTAL TIME:

EXERCISE LOG

	EXERCISE	Sets	Reps	Intensity	1ST SET	2ND SET	3RD SET	4TH SET	5TH SET	REST
1										
2										
3										
4										
5										
6										
7										
8										
9										
10										

MOOD AND ENERGY LEVELS

CARDIO

TYPE	TIME	CALORIES BURNED'

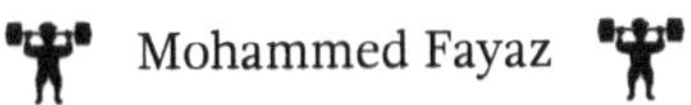

NUTRITION TRACKER

BODY WEIGHT: ___________________________

BODY FAT %: ___________________________

SLEEP (HOURS): ___________________________

SUPPLEMENTS: ___________________________

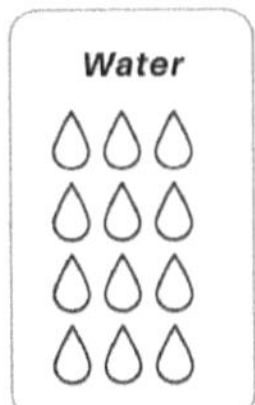

FOOD/MEAL	SERV	CARBS	PROTEIN	FAT	CALS
CALORIES CONSUMED					

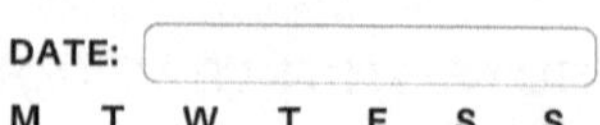 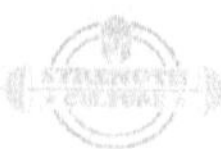

Muscle Mastery

DATE: [ ]

M   T   W   T   F   S   S

DAILY STEPS:

MUSCLE GROUP :

DAILY GOALS :

TOTAL TIME:

EXERCISE LOG

	EXERCISE	Sets	Reps	Intensity	1ST SET	2ND SET	3RD SET	4TH SET	5TH SET	REST
1										
2										
3										
4										
5										
6										
7										
8										
9										
10										

MOOD AND ENERGY LEVELS

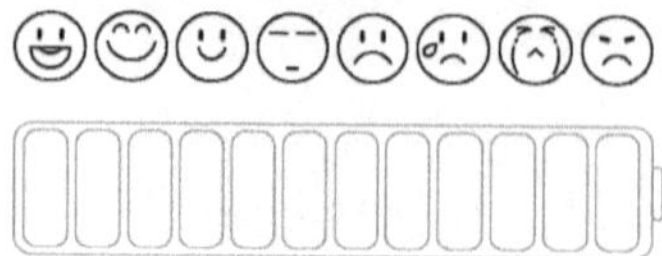

CARDIO

TYPE	TIME	CALORIES BURNED'

NUTRITION TRACKER

BODY WEIGHT: _______________________________

BODY FAT %: _______________________________

SLEEP (HOURS): _______________________________

SUPPLEMENTS: _______________________________

Water

FOOD/MEAL	SERV	CARBS	PROTEIN	FAT	CALS
CALORIES CONSUMED					

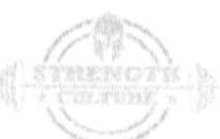

Muscle Mastery

DATE: ____________

M   T   W   T   F   S   S

DAILY STEPS: ____________

MUSCLE GROUP: ____________

DAILY GOALS: ____________

TOTAL TIME: ____________

EXERCISE LOG

	EXERCISE	Sets	Reps	Intensity	1ST SET	2ND SET	3RD SET	4TH SET	5TH SET	REST
1										
2										
3										
4										
5										
6										
7										
8										
9										
10										

MOOD AND ENERGY LEVELS

CARDIO

TYPE	TIME	CALORIES BURNED'

NUTRITION TRACKER

BODY WEIGHT: _______________________________

BODY FAT %: _______________________________

SLEEP (HOURS): _______________________________

SUPPLEMENTS: _______________________________

Water

FOOD/MEAL	SERV	CARBS	PROTEIN	FAT	CALS
CALORIES CONSUMED					

Muscle Mastery

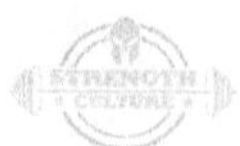

DATE:

M   T   W   T   F   S   S

DAILY STEPS:

MUSCLE GROUP :

DAILY GOALS :

TOTAL TIME:

EXERCISE LOG

	EXERCISE	Sets	Reps	Intensity	1ST SET	2ND SET	3RD SET	4TH SET	5TH SET	REST
1										
2										
3										
4										
5										
6										
7										
8										
9										
10										

MOOD AND ENERGY LEVELS

CARDIO

TYPE	TIME	CALORIES BURNED'

NUTRITION TRACKER

BODY WEIGHT: _______________________________

BODY FAT %: _______________________________

SLEEP (HOURS): _______________________________

SUPPLEMENTS: _______________________________

Water

FOOD/MEAL	SERV	CARBS	PROTEIN	FAT	CALS
CALORIES CONSUMED					

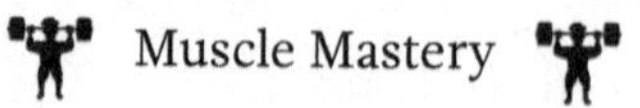

Muscle Mastery

DATE:

M   T   W   T   F   S   S

DAILY STEPS:

MUSCLE GROUP :

DAILY GOALS :

TOTAL TIME:

EXERCISE LOG

	EXERCISE	Sets	Reps	Intensity	1ST SET	2ND SET	3RD SET	4TH SET	5TH SET	REST
1										
2										
3										
4										
5										
6										
7										
8										
9										
10										

MOOD AND ENERGY LEVELS

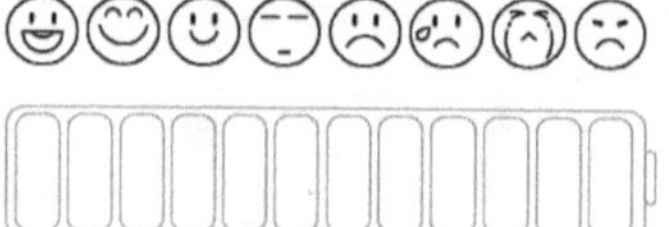

CARDIO

TYPE	TIME	CALORIES BURNED'

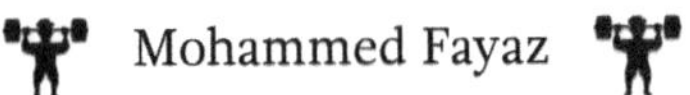

Mohammed Fayaz

NUTRITION TRACKER

BODY WEIGHT: _______________________

BODY FAT %: _______________________

SLEEP (HOURS): _______________________

SUPPLEMENTS: _______________________

Water

FOOD/MEAL	SERV	CARBS	PROTEIN	FAT	CALS
CALORIES CONSUMED					

MONTHLY REFLECTION *Journal*

DATE: **TIME:**

✦ **Monthly Wins**

✦ **How does it make me feel?**

✦ **Challenges**

✦ **How can I improve it?**

Accomplished Goals　**Unaccomplished Goals**　**Goals Next Month**

Habits Retained　**Habits Eliminated**　**New Habits Developed**
(Good & Bad)

Three things that I am most grateful for this month:

Two life lessons I learned this month:

One word that best describes this month:

How will you rate this month? ☆☆☆☆☆

Mohammed Fayaz

DATE: [________________]

M   T   W   T   F   S   S

DAILY STEPS: ____________   **MUSCLE GROUP:** ____________

DAILY GOALS: ____________   **TOTAL TIME:** ____________

EXERCISE LOG

	EXERCISE	Sets	Reps	Intensity	1ST SET	2ND SET	3RD SET	4TH SET	5TH SET	REST
1										
2										
3										
4										
5										
6										
7										
8										
9										
10										

MOOD AND ENERGY LEVELS

CARDIO

TYPE	TIME	CALORIES BURNED'

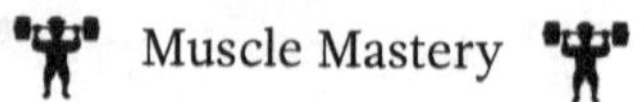

NUTRITION TRACKER

BODY WEIGHT: ___________________________

BODY FAT %: ___________________________

SLEEP (HOURS): ___________________________

SUPPLEMENTS: ___________________________

Water

FOOD/MEAL	SERV	CARBS	PROTEIN	FAT	CALS
CALORIES CONSUMED					

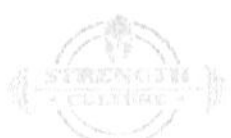 Mohammed Fayaz

DATE: ____________
M T W T F S S

DAILY STEPS: ____________   **MUSCLE GROUP:** ____________

DAILY GOALS: ____________   **TOTAL TIME:** ____________

EXERCISE LOG

	EXERCISE	*Sets*	*Reps*	*Intensity*	*1ST SET*	*2ND SET*	*3RD SET*	*4TH SET*	*5TH SET*	*REST*
1										
2										
3										
4										
5										
6										
7										
8										
9										
10										

MOOD AND ENERGY LEVELS

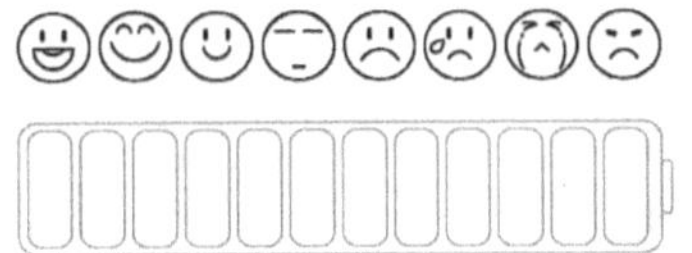

CARDIO

TYPE	TIME	CALORIES BURNED'

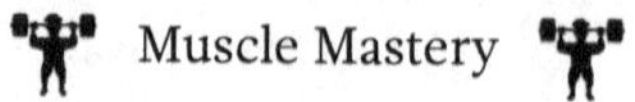 Muscle Mastery

NUTRITION TRACKER

BODY WEIGHT: ______________________

BODY FAT %: ______________________

SLEEP (HOURS): ______________________

SUPPLEMENTS: ______________________

Water

FOOD/MEAL	SERV	CARBS	PROTEIN	FAT	CALS
CALORIES CONSUMED					

DATE:

M   T   W   T   F   S   S

DAILY STEPS:

MUSCLE GROUP:

DAILY GOALS:

TOTAL TIME:

EXERCISE LOG

	EXERCISE	Sets	Reps	Intensity	1ST SET	2ND SET	3RD SET	4TH SET	5TH SET	REST
1										
2										
3										
4										
5										
6										
7										
8										
9										
10										

MOOD AND ENERGY LEVELS

CARDIO

TYPE	TIME	CALORIES BURNED'

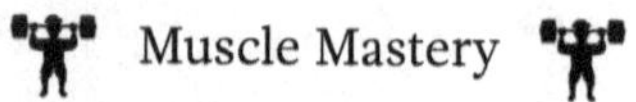

NUTRITION TRACKER

BODY WEIGHT: ______________________________

BODY FAT %: ______________________________

SLEEP (HOURS): ______________________________

SUPPLEMENTS: ______________________________

Water

FOOD/MEAL	SERV	CARBS	PROTEIN	FAT	CALS
CALORIES CONSUMED					

DATE:

M T W T F S S

DAILY STEPS:

MUSCLE GROUP:

DAILY GOALS:

TOTAL TIME:

EXERCISE LOG

	EXERCISE	Sets	Reps	Intensity	1ST SET	2ND SET	3RD SET	4TH SET	5TH SET	REST
1										
2										
3										
4										
5										
6										
7										
8										
9										
10										

MOOD AND ENERGY LEVELS

CARDIO

TYPE	TIME	CALORIES BURNED'

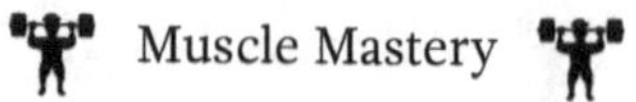

NUTRITION TRACKER

BODY WEIGHT: _______________________

BODY FAT %: _______________________

SLEEP (HOURS): _______________________

SUPPLEMENTS: _______________________

Water

FOOD/MEAL	SERV	CARBS	PROTEIN	FAT	CALS
CALORIES CONSUMED					

DATE:

M   T   W   T   F   S   S

DAILY STEPS:

DAILY GOALS :

MUSCLE GROUP :

TOTAL TIME:

EXERCISE LOG

	EXERCISE	Sets	Reps	Intensity	1ST SET	2ND SET	3RD SET	4TH SET	5TH SET	REST
1										
2										
3										
4										
5										
6										
7										
8										
9										
10										

MOOD AND ENERGY LEVELS

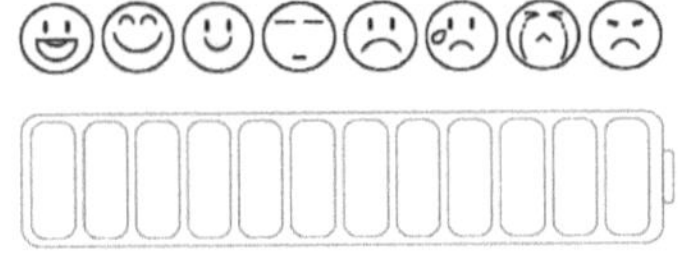

CARDIO

TYPE	TIME	CALORIES BURNED'

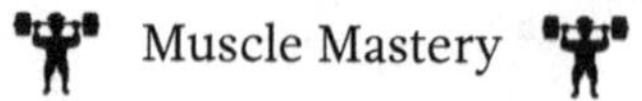

NUTRITION TRACKER

BODY WEIGHT: ___________________________

BODY FAT %: ___________________________

SLEEP (HOURS): ___________________________

SUPPLEMENTS: ___________________________

Water

FOOD/MEAL	SERV	CARBS	PROTEIN	FAT	CALS
CALORIES CONSUMED					

Mohammed Fayaz

DATE:

M T W T F S S

DAILY STEPS:

MUSCLE GROUP:

DAILY GOALS:

TOTAL TIME:

EXERCISE LOG

	EXERCISE	Sets	Reps	Intensity	1ST SET	2ND SET	3RD SET	4TH SET	5TH SET	REST
1										
2										
3										
4										
5										
6										
7										
8										
9										
10										

MOOD AND ENERGY LEVELS

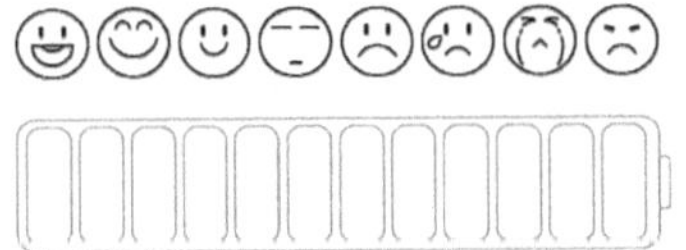

CARDIO

TYPE	TIME	CALORIES BURNED'

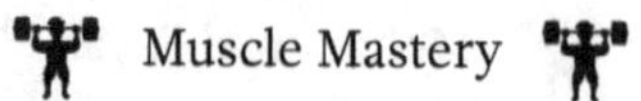

NUTRITION TRACKER

BODY WEIGHT: _______________________________

BODY FAT %: _______________________________

SLEEP (HOURS): _______________________________

SUPPLEMENTS: _______________________________

Water

FOOD/MEAL	SERV	CARBS	PROTEIN	FAT	CALS
CALORIES CONSUMED					

DATE:

M T W T F S S

DAILY STEPS:

MUSCLE GROUP:

DAILY GOALS:

TOTAL TIME:

EXERCISE LOG

	EXERCISE	Sets	Reps	Intensity	1ST SET	2ND SET	3RD SET	4TH SET	5TH SET	REST
1										
2										
3										
4										
5										
6										
7										
8										
9										
10										

MOOD AND ENERGY LEVELS

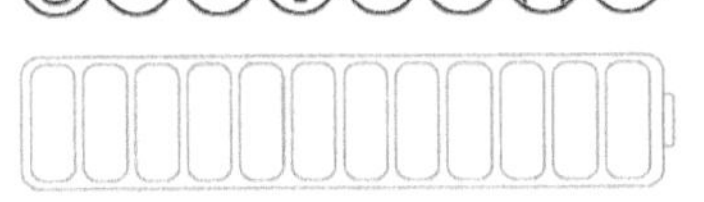

CARDIO

TYPE	TIME	CALORIES BURNED'

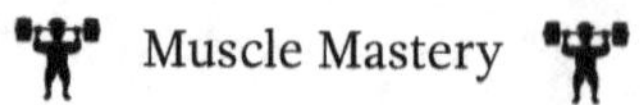

NUTRITION TRACKER

BODY WEIGHT: _______________________

BODY FAT %: _______________________

SLEEP (HOURS): _______________________

SUPPLEMENTS: _______________________

Water

FOOD/MEAL	SERV	CARBS	PROTEIN	FAT	CALS
CALORIES CONSUMED					

Mohammed Fayaz

DATE:

M T W T F S S

DAILY STEPS:

MUSCLE GROUP :

DAILY GOALS :

TOTAL TIME:

EXERCISE LOG

	EXERCISE	Sets	Reps	Intensity	1ST SET	2ND SET	3RD SET	4TH SET	5TH SET	REST
1										
2										
3										
4										
5										
6										
7										
8										
9										
10										

MOOD AND ENERGY LEVELS

CARDIO

TYPE	TIME	CALORIES BURNED'

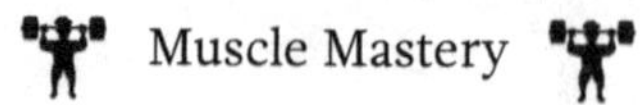

NUTRITION TRACKER

BODY WEIGHT: ______________________________

BODY FAT %: ______________________________

SLEEP (HOURS): ______________________________

SUPPLEMENTS: ______________________________

Water

FOOD/MEAL	SERV	CARBS	PROTEIN	FAT	CALS
CALORIES CONSUMED					

DATE:

M T W T F S S

DAILY STEPS:

MUSCLE GROUP:

DAILY GOALS:

TOTAL TIME:

EXERCISE LOG

	EXERCISE	Sets	Reps	Intensity	1ST SET	2ND SET	3RD SET	4TH SET	5TH SET	REST
1										
2										
3										
4										
5										
6										
7										
8										
9										
10										

MOOD AND ENERGY LEVELS

CARDIO

TYPE	TIME	CALORIES BURNED'

NUTRITION TRACKER

BODY WEIGHT: _______________________________

BODY FAT %: _______________________________

SLEEP (HOURS): _______________________________

SUPPLEMENTS: _______________________________

FOOD/MEAL	SERV	CARBS	PROTEIN	FAT	CALS
CALORIES CONSUMED					

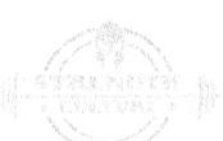

Mohammed Fayaz

DATE:

M   T   W   T   F   S   S

DAILY STEPS:

MUSCLE GROUP:

DAILY GOALS:

TOTAL TIME:

EXERCISE LOG

	EXERCISE	Sets	Reps	Intensity	1ST SET	2ND SET	3RD SET	4TH SET	5TH SET	REST
1										
2										
3										
4										
5										
6										
7										
8										
9										
10										

MOOD AND ENERGY LEVELS

CARDIO

TYPE	TIME	CALORIES BURNED'

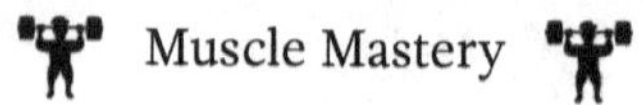

NUTRITION TRACKER

BODY WEIGHT: _______________________

BODY FAT %: _______________________

SLEEP (HOURS): _______________________

SUPPLEMENTS: _______________________

Water

FOOD/MEAL	SERV	CARBS	PROTEIN	FAT	CALS
CALORIES CONSUMED					

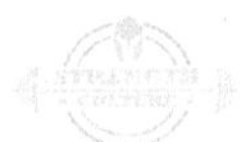 Mohammed Fayaz

DATE: [____________]

M   T   W   T   F   S   S

DAILY STEPS: ________________

MUSCLE GROUP : ________________

DAILY GOALS : ________________

TOTAL TIME: ________________

EXERCISE LOG

	EXERCISE	Sets	Reps	Intensity	1ST SET	2ND SET	3RD SET	4TH SET	5TH SET	REST
1										
2										
3										
4										
5										
6										
7										
8										
9										
10										

MOOD AND ENERGY LEVELS

CARDIO

TYPE	TIME	CALORIES BURNED'

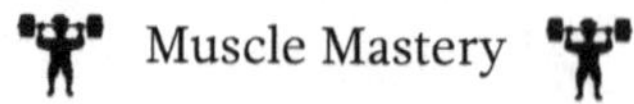 Muscle Mastery

NUTRITION TRACKER

BODY WEIGHT: ______________________

BODY FAT %: ______________________

SLEEP (HOURS): ______________________

SUPPLEMENTS: ______________________

FOOD/MEAL	SERV	CARBS	PROTEIN	FAT	CALS
CALORIES CONSUMED					

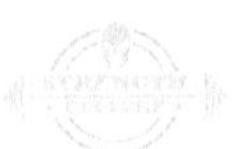 Mohammed Fayaz

DATE:

M   T   W   T   F   S   S

DAILY STEPS:

MUSCLE GROUP :

DAILY GOALS :

TOTAL TIME:

EXERCISE LOG

	EXERCISE	Sets	Reps	Intensity	1ST SET	2ND SET	3RD SET	4TH SET	5TH SET	REST
1										
2										
3										
4										
5										
6										
7										
8										
9										
10										

MOOD AND ENERGY LEVELS

CARDIO

TYPE	TIME	CALORIES BURNED'

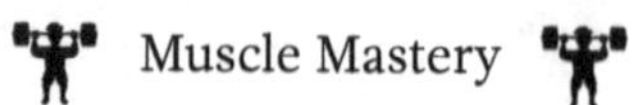

NUTRITION TRACKER

BODY WEIGHT: _______________________________

BODY FAT %: _______________________________

SLEEP (HOURS): _______________________________

SUPPLEMENTS: _______________________________

Water

FOOD/MEAL	SERV	CARBS	PROTEIN	FAT	CALS
CALORIES CONSUMED					

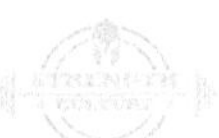

Mohammed Fayaz

DATE: [ ]

M T W T F S S

DAILY STEPS:

MUSCLE GROUP :

DAILY GOALS :

TOTAL TIME:

EXERCISE LOG

	EXERCISE	Sets	Reps	Intensity	1ST SET	2ND SET	3RD SET	4TH SET	5TH SET	REST
1										
2										
3										
4										
5										
6										
7										
8										
9										
10										

MOOD AND ENERGY LEVELS

CARDIO

TYPE	TIME	CALORIES BURNED'

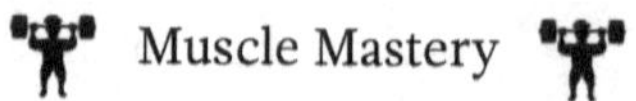

NUTRITION TRACKER

BODY WEIGHT: ______________________________

BODY FAT %: ______________________________

SLEEP (HOURS): ______________________________

SUPPLEMENTS: ______________________________

Water

FOOD/MEAL	SERV	CARBS	PROTEIN	FAT	CALS
CALORIES CONSUMED					

Mohammed Fayaz

DATE:

M T W T F S S

DAILY STEPS:

MUSCLE GROUP :

DAILY GOALS :

TOTAL TIME:

EXERCISE LOG

	EXERCISE	Sets	Reps	Intensity	1ST SET	2ND SET	3RD SET	4TH SET	5TH SET	REST
1										
2										
3										
4										
5										
6										
7										
8										
9										
10										

MOOD AND ENERGY LEVELS

CARDIO

TYPE	TIME	CALORIES BURNED'

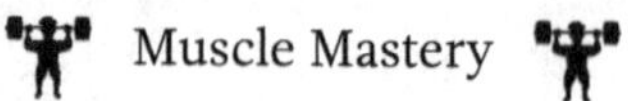

NUTRITION TRACKER

BODY WEIGHT: _______________________

BODY FAT %: _______________________

SLEEP (HOURS): _______________________

SUPPLEMENTS: _______________________

Water

FOOD/MEAL	SERV	CARBS	PROTEIN	FAT	CALS
CALORIES CONSUMED					

Mohammed Fayaz

DATE: __________

M T W T F S S

DAILY STEPS: __________

DAILY GOALS: __________

MUSCLE GROUP: __________

TOTAL TIME: __________

EXERCISE LOG

	EXERCISE	Sets	Reps	Intensity	1ST SET	2ND SET	3RD SET	4TH SET	5TH SET	REST
1										
2										
3										
4										
5										
6										
7										
8										
9										
10										

MOOD AND ENERGY LEVELS

CARDIO

TYPE	TIME	CALORIES BURNED'

NUTRITION TRACKER

BODY WEIGHT: _______________________

BODY FAT %: _______________________

SLEEP (HOURS): _______________________

SUPPLEMENTS: _______________________

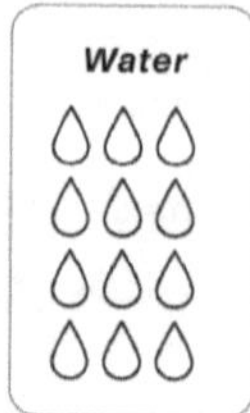

FOOD/MEAL	SERV	CARBS	PROTEIN	FAT	CALS
CALORIES CONSUMED					

DATE:

M T W T F S S

DAILY STEPS:

MUSCLE GROUP:

DAILY GOALS:

TOTAL TIME:

EXERCISE LOG

	EXERCISE	Sets	Reps	Intensity	1ST SET	2ND SET	3RD SET	4TH SET	5TH SET	REST
1										
2										
3										
4										
5										
6										
7										
8										
9										
10										

MOOD AND ENERGY LEVELS

CARDIO

TYPE	TIME	CALORIES BURNED'

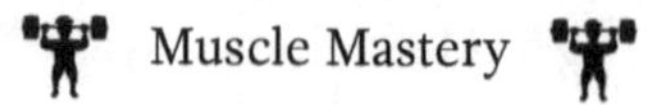 Muscle Mastery

NUTRITION TRACKER

BODY WEIGHT: _______________________

BODY FAT %: _______________________

SLEEP (HOURS): _______________________

SUPPLEMENTS: _______________________

Water

FOOD/MEAL	SERV	CARBS	PROTEIN	FAT	CALS
CALORIES CONSUMED					

🏋 **Mohammed Fayaz** 🏋

DATE: ______________

M   T   W   T   F   S   S

DAILY STEPS: ____________________   **MUSCLE GROUP:** ____________________

DAILY GOALS: ____________________   **TOTAL TIME:** ____________________

EXERCISE LOG

	EXERCISE	Sets	Reps	Intensity	1ST SET	2ND SET	3RD SET	4TH SET	5TH SET	REST
1										
2										
3										
4										
5										
6										
7										
8										
9										
10										

MOOD AND ENERGY LEVELS

CARDIO

TYPE	TIME	CALORIES BURNED'

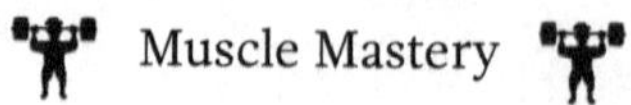

NUTRITION TRACKER

BODY WEIGHT: _______________________

BODY FAT %: _______________________

SLEEP (HOURS): _______________________

SUPPLEMENTS: _______________________

Water

FOOD/MEAL	SERV	CARBS	PROTEIN	FAT	CALS
CALORIES CONSUMED					

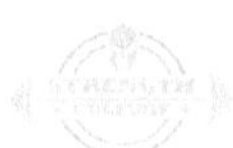 Mohammed Fayaz

DATE: [ ]

M T W T F S S

DAILY STEPS: ________________   **MUSCLE GROUP:** ________________

DAILY GOALS: ________________   **TOTAL TIME:** ________________

EXERCISE LOG

	EXERCISE	Sets	Reps	Intensity	1ST SET	2ND SET	3RD SET	4TH SET	5TH SET	REST
1										
2										
3										
4										
5										
6										
7										
8										
9										
10										

MOOD AND ENERGY LEVELS

CARDIO

TYPE	TIME	CALORIES BURNED'

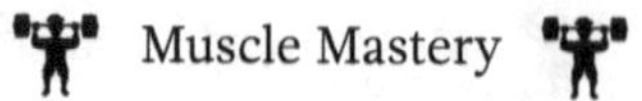

NUTRITION TRACKER

BODY WEIGHT: ___________________________

BODY FAT %: ___________________________

SLEEP (HOURS): ___________________________

SUPPLEMENTS: ___________________________

Water

FOOD/MEAL	SERV	CARBS	PROTEIN	FAT	CALS
CALORIES CONSUMED					

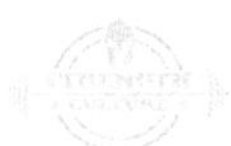 Mohammed Fayaz

DATE:

M T W T F S S

DAILY STEPS:

MUSCLE GROUP :

DAILY GOALS :

TOTAL TIME:

EXERCISE LOG

	EXERCISE	Sets	Reps	Intensity	1ST SET	2ND SET	3RD SET	4TH SET	5TH SET	REST
1										
2										
3										
4										
5										
6										
7										
8										
9										
10										

MOOD AND ENERGY LEVELS

CARDIO

TYPE	TIME	CALORIES BURNED'

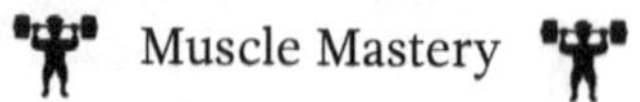

NUTRITION TRACKER

BODY WEIGHT: _______________________

BODY FAT %: _______________________

SLEEP (HOURS): _______________________

SUPPLEMENTS: _______________________

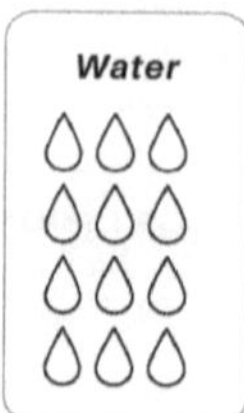

FOOD/MEAL	SERV	CARBS	PROTEIN	FAT	CALS
CALORIES CONSUMED					

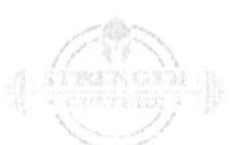 Mohammed Fayaz

DATE:

M T W T F S S

DAILY STEPS:

MUSCLE GROUP:

DAILY GOALS:

TOTAL TIME:

EXERCISE LOG

	EXERCISE	Sets	Reps	Intensity	1ST SET	2ND SET	3RD SET	4TH SET	5TH SET	REST
1										
2										
3										
4										
5										
6										
7										
8										
9										
10										

MOOD AND ENERGY LEVELS

CARDIO

TYPE	TIME	CALORIES BURNED'

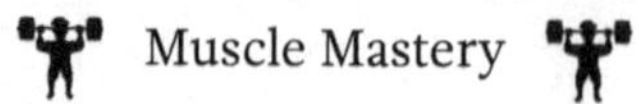

NUTRITION TRACKER

BODY WEIGHT: _______________________

BODY FAT %: _______________________

SLEEP (HOURS): _______________________

SUPPLEMENTS: _______________________

Water

FOOD/MEAL	SERV	CARBS	PROTEIN	FAT	CALS
CALORIES CONSUMED					

DATE:

M T W T F S S

DAILY STEPS:

MUSCLE GROUP:

DAILY GOALS:

TOTAL TIME:

EXERCISE LOG

	EXERCISE	Sets	Reps	Intensity	1ST SET	2ND SET	3RD SET	4TH SET	5TH SET	REST
1										
2										
3										
4										
5										
6										
7										
8										
9										
10										

MOOD AND ENERGY LEVELS

CARDIO

TYPE	TIME	CALORIES BURNED'

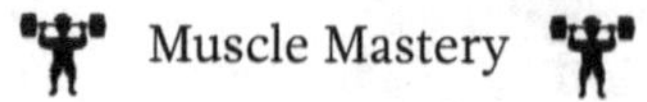

NUTRITION TRACKER

BODY WEIGHT: _______________________

BODY FAT %: _______________________

SLEEP (HOURS): _______________________

SUPPLEMENTS: _______________________

Water

FOOD/MEAL	SERV	CARBS	PROTEIN	FAT	CALS
CALORIES CONSUMED					

Mohammed Fayaz

DATE: [　　　　　　　　　]

M   T   W   T   F   S   S

DAILY STEPS:

MUSCLE GROUP:

DAILY GOALS:

TOTAL TIME:

EXERCISE LOG

	EXERCISE	Sets	Reps	Intensity	1ST SET	2ND SET	3RD SET	4TH SET	5TH SET	REST
1										
2										
3										
4										
5										
6										
7										
8										
9										
10										

MOOD AND ENERGY LEVELS

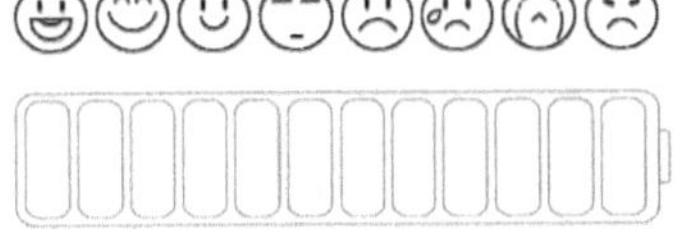

CARDIO

TYPE	TIME	CALORIES BURNED'

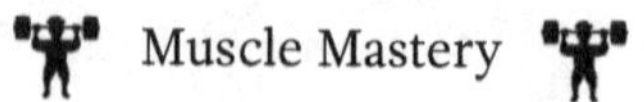 **Muscle Mastery**

NUTRITION TRACKER

BODY WEIGHT: _______________________

BODY FAT %: _______________________

SLEEP (HOURS): _______________________

SUPPLEMENTS: _______________________

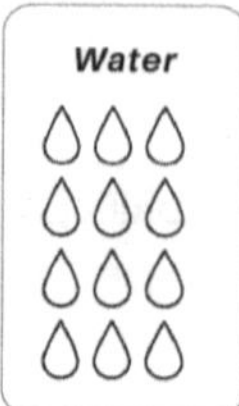

FOOD/MEAL	SERV	CARBS	PROTEIN	FAT	CALS
CALORIES CONSUMED					

Mohammed Fayaz

DATE:

M T W T F S S

DAILY STEPS:

MUSCLE GROUP:

DAILY GOALS:

TOTAL TIME:

EXERCISE LOG

	EXERCISE	Sets	Reps	Intensity	1ST SET	2ND SET	3RD SET	4TH SET	5TH SET	REST
1										
2										
3										
4										
5										
6										
7										
8										
9										
10										

MOOD AND ENERGY LEVELS

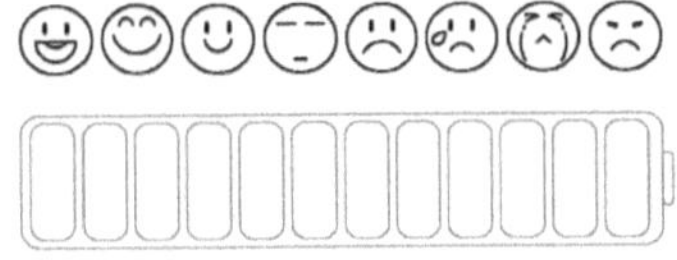

CARDIO

TYPE	TIME	CALORIES BURNED'

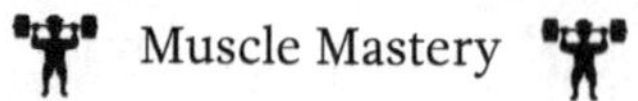

NUTRITION TRACKER

BODY WEIGHT: ______________________________

BODY FAT %: ______________________________

SLEEP (HOURS): ______________________________

SUPPLEMENTS: ______________________________

Water

FOOD/MEAL	SERV	CARBS	PROTEIN	FAT	CALS
CALORIES CONSUMED					

DATE:

M   T   W   T   F   S   S

DAILY STEPS:

MUSCLE GROUP:

DAILY GOALS:

TOTAL TIME:

EXERCISE LOG

	EXERCISE	Sets	Reps	Intensity	1ST SET	2ND SET	3RD SET	4TH SET	5TH SET	REST
1										
2										
3										
4										
5										
6										
7										
8										
9										
10										

MOOD AND ENERGY LEVELS

CARDIO

TYPE	TIME	CALORIES BURNED'

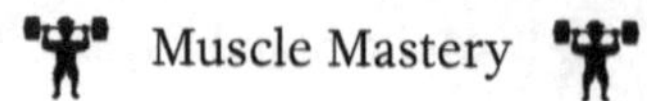

NUTRITION TRACKER

BODY WEIGHT: _______________________________

BODY FAT %: _______________________________

SLEEP (HOURS): _______________________________

SUPPLEMENTS: _______________________________

Water

FOOD/MEAL	SERV	CARBS	PROTEIN	FAT	CALS
CALORIES CONSUMED					

Mohammed Fayaz

DATE:

M T W T F S S

DAILY STEPS:

MUSCLE GROUP:

DAILY GOALS:

TOTAL TIME:

EXERCISE LOG

	EXERCISE	Sets	Reps	Intensity	1ST SET	2ND SET	3RD SET	4TH SET	5TH SET	REST
1										
2										
3										
4										
5										
6										
7										
8										
9										
10										

MOOD AND ENERGY LEVELS

CARDIO

TYPE	TIME	CALORIES BURNED'

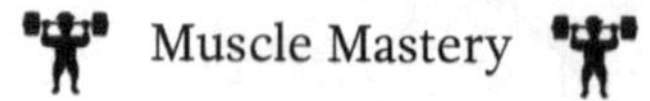

NUTRITION TRACKER

BODY WEIGHT: _______________________________

BODY FAT %: _______________________________

SLEEP (HOURS): _______________________________

SUPPLEMENTS: _______________________________

Water

FOOD/MEAL	SERV	CARBS	PROTEIN	FAT	CALS
CALORIES CONSUMED					

DATE:

M   T   W   T   F   S   S

DAILY STEPS:

MUSCLE GROUP:

DAILY GOALS:

TOTAL TIME:

EXERCISE LOG

	EXERCISE	Sets	Reps	Intensity	1ST SET	2ND SET	3RD SET	4TH SET	5TH SET	REST
1										
2										
3										
4										
5										
6										
7										
8										
9										
10										

MOOD AND ENERGY LEVELS

CARDIO

TYPE	TIME	CALORIES BURNED'

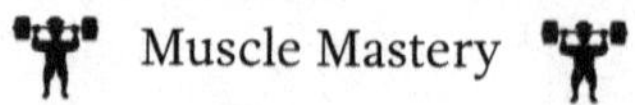

NUTRITION TRACKER

BODY WEIGHT: _______________________

BODY FAT %: _______________________

SLEEP (HOURS): _______________________

SUPPLEMENTS: _______________________

Water

FOOD/MEAL	SERV	CARBS	PROTEIN	FAT	CALS
CALORIES CONSUMED					

Mohammed Fayaz

DATE:

M T W T F S S

DAILY STEPS:

MUSCLE GROUP:

DAILY GOALS:

TOTAL TIME:

EXERCISE LOG

	EXERCISE	Sets	Reps	Intensity	1ST SET	2ND SET	3RD SET	4TH SET	5TH SET	REST
1										
2										
3										
4										
5										
6										
7										
8										
9										
10										

MOOD AND ENERGY LEVELS

CARDIO

TYPE	TIME	CALORIES BURNED'

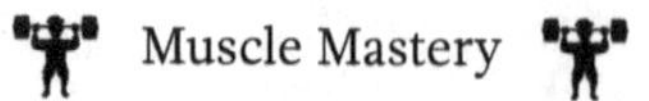 Muscle Mastery

NUTRITION TRACKER

BODY WEIGHT:

BODY FAT %:

SLEEP (HOURS):

SUPPLEMENTS:

FOOD/MEAL	SERV	CARBS	PROTEIN	FAT	CALS
CALORIES CONSUMED					

Mohammed Fayaz

DATE: [ ]

M   T   W   T   F   S   S

DAILY STEPS:

MUSCLE GROUP:

DAILY GOALS:

TOTAL TIME:

EXERCISE LOG

	EXERCISE	Sets	Reps	Intensity	1ST SET	2ND SET	3RD SET	4TH SET	5TH SET	REST
1										
2										
3										
4										
5										
6										
7										
8										
9										
10										

MOOD AND ENERGY LEVELS

CARDIO

TYPE	TIME	CALORIES BURNED'

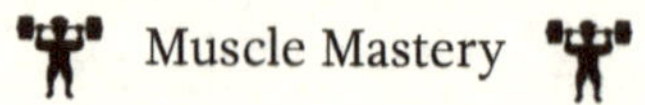 Muscle Mastery

NUTRITION TRACKER

BODY WEIGHT: _______________________________

BODY FAT %: _______________________________

SLEEP (HOURS): _______________________________

SUPPLEMENTS: _______________________________

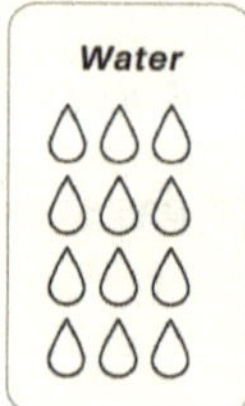

FOOD/MEAL	SERV	CARBS	PROTEIN	FAT	CALS
CALORIES CONSUMED					

DATE:

M   T   W   T   F   S   S

DAILY STEPS:

MUSCLE GROUP:

DAILY GOALS:

TOTAL TIME:

EXERCISE LOG

	EXERCISE	Sets	Reps	Intensity	1ST SET	2ND SET	3RD SET	4TH SET	5TH SET	REST
1										
2										
3										
4										
5										
6										
7										
8										
9										
10										

MOOD AND ENERGY LEVELS

CARDIO

TYPE	TIME	CALORIES BURNED'

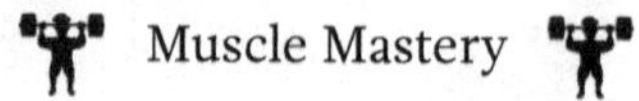

NUTRITION TRACKER

BODY WEIGHT: ______________________

BODY FAT %: ______________________

SLEEP (HOURS): ______________________

SUPPLEMENTS: ______________________

Water

FOOD/MEAL	SERV	CARBS	PROTEIN	FAT	CALS
CALORIES CONSUMED					

DATE:

M T W T F S S

DAILY STEPS:

MUSCLE GROUP:

DAILY GOALS :

TOTAL TIME:

EXERCISE LOG

	EXERCISE	Sets	Reps	Intensity	1ST SET	2ND SET	3RD SET	4TH SET	5TH SET	REST
1										
2										
3										
4										
5										
6										
7										
8										
9										
10										

MOOD AND ENERGY LEVELS

CARDIO

TYPE	TIME	CALORIES BURNED'

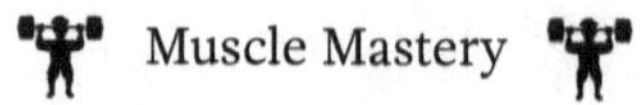

NUTRITION TRACKER

BODY WEIGHT: _______________________

BODY FAT %: _______________________

SLEEP (HOURS): _______________________

SUPPLEMENTS: _______________________

Water

FOOD/MEAL	SERV	CARBS	PROTEIN	FAT	CALS
CALORIES CONSUMED					

MONTHLY REFLECTION *Journal*

DATE: TIME:

✦ **Monthly Wins**

✦ **How does it make me feel?**

✦ **Challenges**

✦ **How can I improve it?**

Accomplished Goals **Unaccomplished Goals** **Goals Next Month**

Habits Retained **Habits Eliminated** **New Habits Developed**
(Good & Bad)

Three things that I am most grateful for this month:

Two life lessons I learned this month:

One word that best describes this month:

How will you rate this month? ☆☆☆☆☆

Muscle Mastery 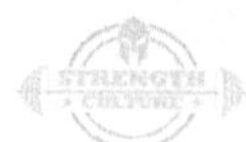

DATE:

M T W T F S S

DAILY STEPS:

MUSCLE GROUP:

DAILY GOALS:

TOTAL TIME:

EXERCISE LOG

	EXERCISE	Sets	Reps	Intensity	1ST SET	2ND SET	3RD SET	4TH SET	5TH SET	REST
1										
2										
3										
4										
5										
6										
7										
8										
9										
10										

MOOD AND ENERGY LEVELS

CARDIO

TYPE	TIME	CALORIES BURNED'

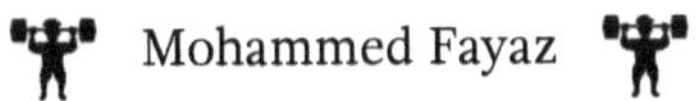

NUTRITION TRACKER

BODY WEIGHT: _______________________________

BODY FAT %: _______________________________

SLEEP (HOURS): _______________________________

SUPPLEMENTS: _______________________________

Water

FOOD/MEAL	SERV	CARBS	PROTEIN	FAT	CALS
CALORIES CONSUMED				

Muscle Mastery

DATE:

M   T   W   T   F   S   S

DAILY STEPS:

DAILY GOALS:

MUSCLE GROUP:

TOTAL TIME:

EXERCISE LOG

	EXERCISE	Sets	Reps	Intensity	1ST SET	2ND SET	3RD SET	4TH SET	5TH SET	REST
1										
2										
3										
4										
5										
6										
7										
8										
9										
10										

MOOD AND ENERGY LEVELS

CARDIO

TYPE	TIME	CALORIES BURNED'

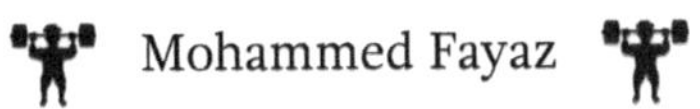

NUTRITION TRACKER

BODY WEIGHT: ___________________________

BODY FAT %: ___________________________

SLEEP (HOURS): ___________________________

SUPPLEMENTS: ___________________________

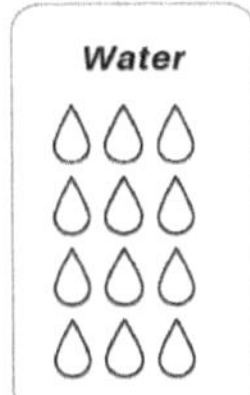

FOOD/MEAL	SERV	CARBS	PROTEIN	FAT	CALS
CALORIES CONSUMED					

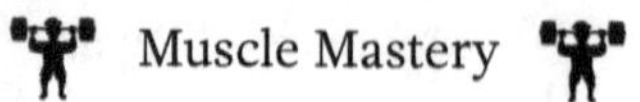 Muscle Mastery

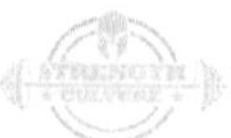

DATE: ____________

M T W T F S S

DAILY STEPS: ______________   **MUSCLE GROUP:** ______________

DAILY GOALS: ______________   **TOTAL TIME:** ______________

EXERCISE LOG

	EXERCISE	Sets	Reps	Intensity	1ST SET	2ND SET	3RD SET	4TH SET	5TH SET	REST
1										
2										
3										
4										
5										
6										
7										
8										
9										
10										

MOOD AND ENERGY LEVELS

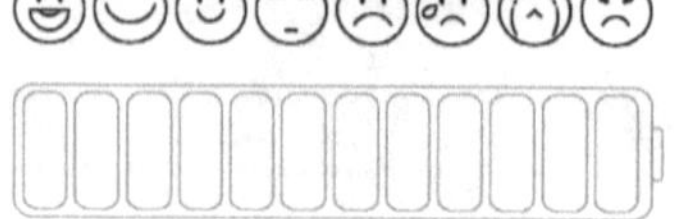

CARDIO

TYPE	TIME	CALORIES BURNED'

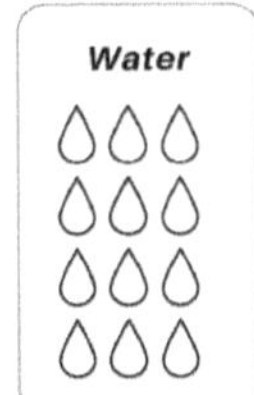

NUTRITION TRACKER

BODY WEIGHT: ___________________________

BODY FAT %: ___________________________

SLEEP (HOURS): ___________________________

SUPPLEMENTS: ___________________________

Water

FOOD/MEAL	SERV	CARBS	PROTEIN	FAT	CALS
CALORIES CONSUMED					

Muscle Mastery 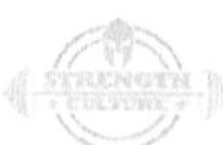

DATE:

M T W T F S S

DAILY STEPS:

MUSCLE GROUP :

DAILY GOALS :

TOTAL TIME:

EXERCISE LOG

	EXERCISE	Sets	Reps	Intensity	1ST SET	2ND SET	3RD SET	4TH SET	5TH SET	REST
1										
2										
3										
4										
5										
6										
7										
8										
9										
10										

MOOD AND ENERGY LEVELS

CARDIO

TYPE	TIME	CALORIES BURNED'

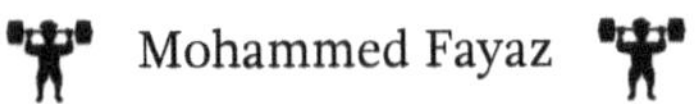 Mohammed Fayaz

NUTRITION TRACKER

BODY WEIGHT: ______________________________

BODY FAT %: ______________________________

SLEEP (HOURS): ______________________________

SUPPLEMENTS: ______________________________

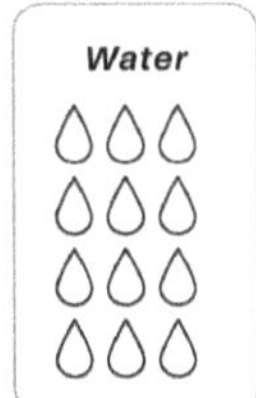

FOOD/MEAL	SERV	CARBS	PROTEIN	FAT	CALS
CALORIES CONSUMED					

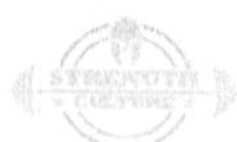# Muscle Mastery

DATE: ____________

M   T   W   T   F   S   S

DAILY STEPS: ________________

MUSCLE GROUP: ________________

DAILY GOALS: ________________

TOTAL TIME: ________________

EXERCISE LOG

	EXERCISE	Sets	Reps	Intensity	1ST SET	2ND SET	3RD SET	4TH SET	5TH SET	REST
1										
2										
3										
4										
5										
6										
7										
8										
9										
10										

MOOD AND ENERGY LEVELS

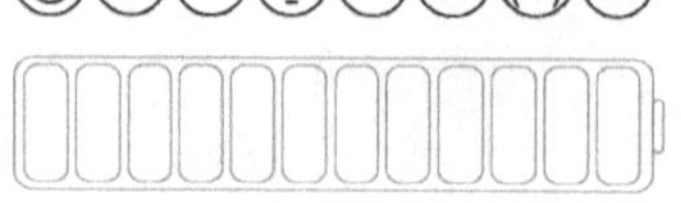

CARDIO

TYPE	TIME	CALORIES BURNED'

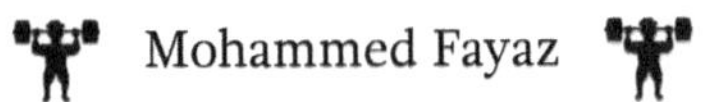

NUTRITION TRACKER

BODY WEIGHT: ___________________________

BODY FAT %: ___________________________

SLEEP (HOURS): ___________________________

SUPPLEMENTS: ___________________________

Water

FOOD/MEAL	SERV	CARBS	PROTEIN	FAT	CALS
CALORIES CONSUMED					

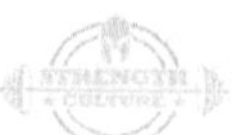

Muscle Mastery

DATE: [   ]

M T W T F S S

DAILY STEPS: ___________________

MUSCLE GROUP : ___________________

DAILY GOALS : ___________________

TOTAL TIME: ___________________

EXERCISE LOG

	EXERCISE	Sets	Reps	Intensity	1ST SET	2ND SET	3RD SET	4TH SET	5TH SET	REST
1										
2										
3										
4										
5										
6										
7										
8										
9										
10										

MOOD AND ENERGY LEVELS

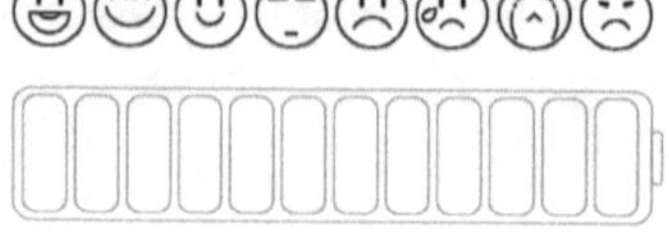

CARDIO

TYPE	TIME	CALORIES BURNED'

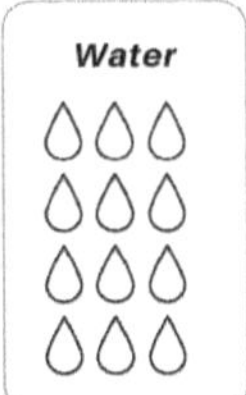

Mohammed Fayaz

NUTRITION TRACKER

BODY WEIGHT: ______________________

BODY FAT %: ______________________

SLEEP (HOURS): ______________________

SUPPLEMENTS: ______________________

Water

FOOD/MEAL	SERV	CARBS	PROTEIN	FAT	CALS
CALORIES CONSUMED					

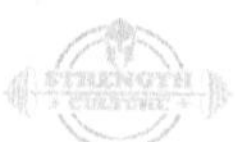

Muscle Mastery

DATE: [ ]

M T W T F S S

DAILY STEPS: _______________   **MUSCLE GROUP:** _______________

DAILY GOALS: _______________   **TOTAL TIME:** _______________

EXERCISE LOG

	EXERCISE	Sets	Reps	Intensity	1ST SET	2ND SET	3RD SET	4TH SET	5TH SET	REST
1										
2										
3										
4										
5										
6										
7										
8										
9										
10										

MOOD AND ENERGY LEVELS

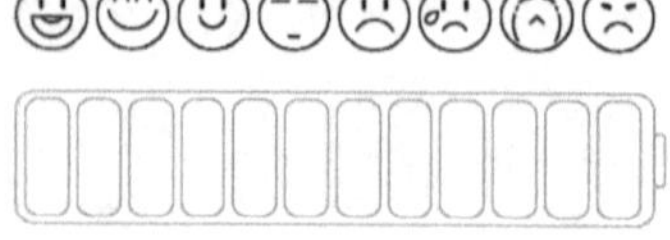

CARDIO

TYPE	TIME	CALORIES BURNED'

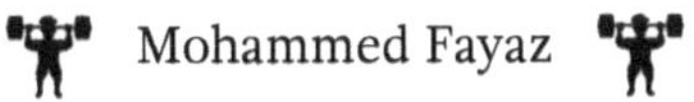

NUTRITION TRACKER

BODY WEIGHT: _______________________________

BODY FAT %: _______________________________

SLEEP (HOURS): _______________________________

SUPPLEMENTS: _______________________________

Water

FOOD/MEAL	SERV	CARBS	PROTEIN	FAT	CALS
CALORIES CONSUMED					

 Muscle Mastery

DATE: ____________
M T W T F S S

DAILY STEPS: ______________   **MUSCLE GROUP:** ______________

DAILY GOALS: ______________   **TOTAL TIME:** ______________

EXERCISE LOG

	EXERCISE	Sets	Reps	Intensity	1ST SET	2ND SET	3RD SET	4TH SET	5TH SET	REST
1										
2										
3										
4										
5										
6										
7										
8										
9										
10										

MOOD AND ENERGY LEVELS

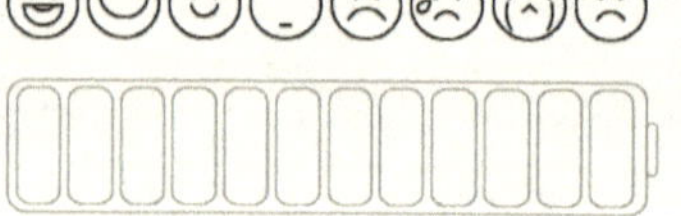

CARDIO

TYPE	TIME	CALORIES BURNED'

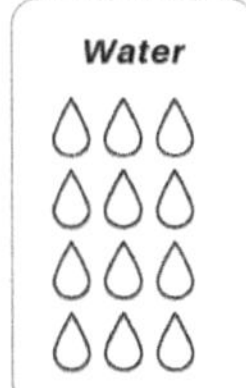

Mohammed Fayaz

NUTRITION TRACKER

BODY WEIGHT: _______________________

BODY FAT %: _______________________

SLEEP (HOURS): _______________________

SUPPLEMENTS: _______________________

Water

FOOD/MEAL	SERV	CARBS	PROTEIN	FAT	CALS
CALORIES CONSUMED					

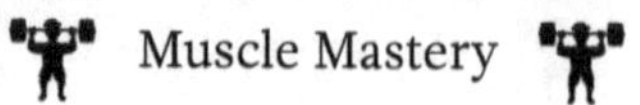
Muscle Mastery

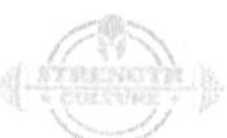

DATE: [　　　　　　　　　]

M　T　W　T　F　S　S

DAILY STEPS: __________________

MUSCLE GROUP : __________________

DAILY GOALS : __________________

TOTAL TIME: __________________

EXERCISE LOG

	EXERCISE	Sets	Reps	Intensity	1ST SET	2ND SET	3RD SET	4TH SET	5TH SET	REST
1										
2										
3										
4										
5										
6										
7										
8										
9										
10										

MOOD AND ENERGY LEVELS

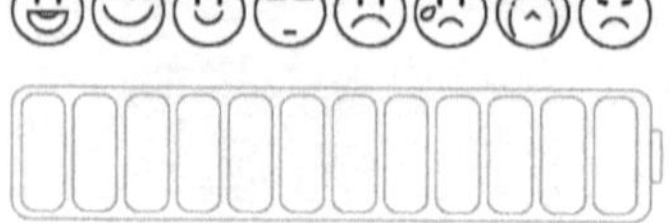

CARDIO

TYPE	TIME	CALORIES BURNED'

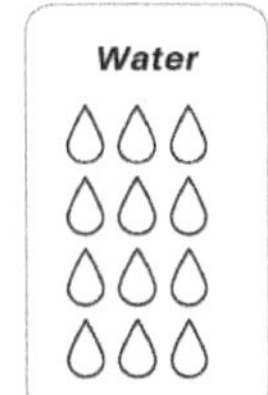

Mohammed Fayaz

NUTRITION TRACKER

BODY WEIGHT: _______________________

BODY FAT %: _______________________

SLEEP (HOURS): _______________________

SUPPLEMENTS: _______________________

FOOD/MEAL	SERV	CARBS	PROTEIN	FAT	CALS
CALORIES CONSUMED					

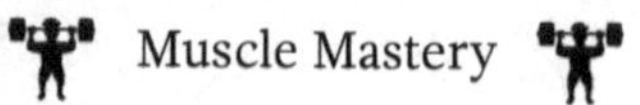 **Muscle Mastery**

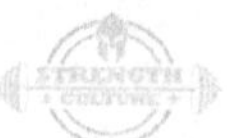

DATE: __________________

M T W T F S S

DAILY STEPS: ______________________

MUSCLE GROUP: ______________________

DAILY GOALS: ______________________

TOTAL TIME: ______________________

EXERCISE LOG

	EXERCISE	Sets	Reps	Intensity	1ST SET	2ND SET	3RD SET	4TH SET	5TH SET	REST
1										
2										
3										
4										
5										
6										
7										
8										
9										
10										

MOOD AND ENERGY LEVELS

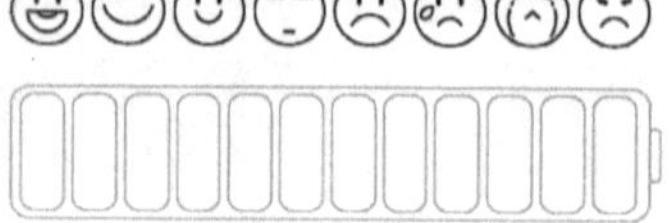

CARDIO

TYPE	TIME	CALORIES BURNED'

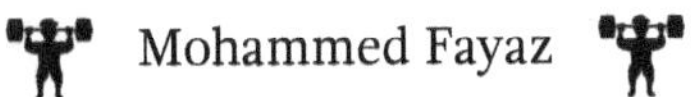

NUTRITION TRACKER

BODY WEIGHT: _______________________

BODY FAT %: _______________________

SLEEP (HOURS): _______________________

SUPPLEMENTS: _______________________

Water

FOOD/MEAL	SERV	CARBS	PROTEIN	FAT	CALS
CALORIES CONSUMED					

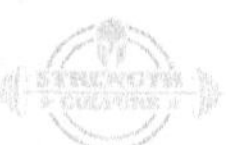

Muscle Mastery

DATE:

M T W T F S S

DAILY STEPS:

DAILY GOALS:

MUSCLE GROUP:

TOTAL TIME:

EXERCISE LOG

	EXERCISE	Sets	Reps	Intensity	1ST SET	2ND SET	3RD SET	4TH SET	5TH SET	REST
1										
2										
3										
4										
5										
6										
7										
8										
9										
10										

MOOD AND ENERGY LEVELS

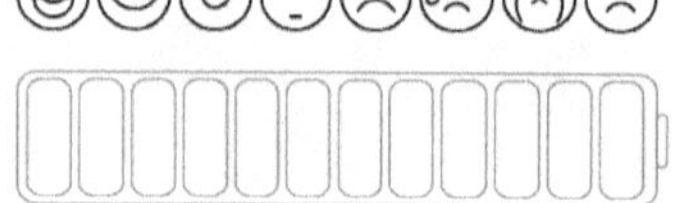

CARDIO

TYPE	TIME	CALORIES BURNED'

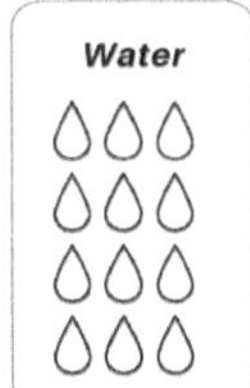

NUTRITION TRACKER

BODY WEIGHT: _______________________________

BODY FAT %: _______________________________

SLEEP (HOURS): _______________________________

SUPPLEMENTS: _______________________________

Water

FOOD/MEAL	SERV	CARBS	PROTEIN	FAT	CALS
CALORIES CONSUMED					

Muscle Mastery

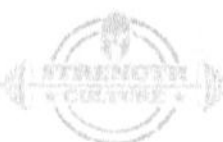

DATE:

M T W T F S S

DAILY STEPS:

DAILY GOALS :

MUSCLE GROUP :

TOTAL TIME:

EXERCISE LOG

	EXERCISE	Sets	Reps	Intensity	1ST SET	2ND SET	3RD SET	4TH SET	5TH SET	REST
1										
2										
3										
4										
5										
6										
7										
8										
9										
10										

MOOD AND ENERGY LEVELS

CARDIO

TYPE	TIME	CALORIES BURNED'

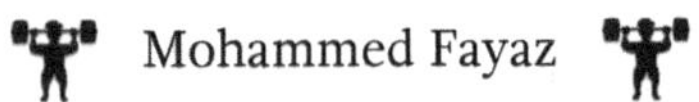

NUTRITION TRACKER

BODY WEIGHT: ___________________________

BODY FAT %: ___________________________

SLEEP (HOURS): ___________________________

SUPPLEMENTS: ___________________________

Water

FOOD/MEAL	SERV	CARBS	PROTEIN	FAT	CALS
CALORIES CONSUMED					

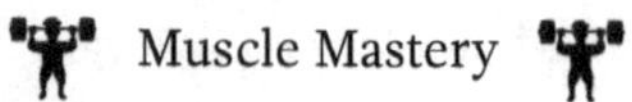 Muscle Mastery 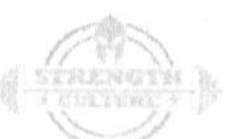

DATE: [ ]

M   T   W   T   F   S   S

DAILY STEPS: __________

MUSCLE GROUP: __________

DAILY GOALS: __________

TOTAL TIME: __________

EXERCISE LOG

	EXERCISE	Sets	Reps	Intensity	1ST SET	2ND SET	3RD SET	4TH SET	5TH SET	REST
1										
2										
3										
4										
5										
6										
7										
8										
9										
10										

MOOD AND ENERGY LEVELS

CARDIO

TYPE	TIME	CALORIES BURNED'

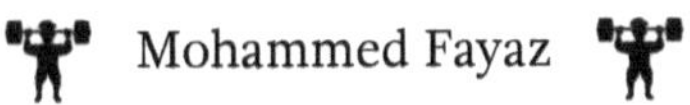

NUTRITION TRACKER

BODY WEIGHT: ___________________________

BODY FAT %: ___________________________

SLEEP (HOURS): ___________________________

SUPPLEMENTS: ___________________________

Water

FOOD/MEAL	SERV	CARBS	PROTEIN	FAT	CALS
CALORIES CONSUMED					

Muscle Mastery 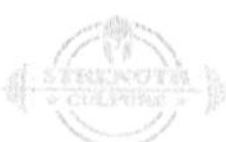

DATE: ________________

M T W T F S S

DAILY STEPS: ________________

MUSCLE GROUP: ________________

DAILY GOALS: ________________

TOTAL TIME: ________________

EXERCISE LOG

	EXERCISE	Sets	Reps	Intensity	1ST SET	2ND SET	3RD SET	4TH SET	5TH SET	REST
1										
2										
3										
4										
5										
6										
7										
8										
9										
10										

MOOD AND ENERGY LEVELS

CARDIO

TYPE	TIME	CALORIES BURNED'

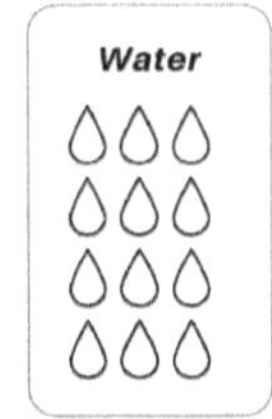

Mohammed Fayaz

NUTRITION TRACKER

BODY WEIGHT: _______________________

BODY FAT %: _______________________

SLEEP (HOURS): _______________________

SUPPLEMENTS: _______________________

Water

FOOD/MEAL	SERV	CARBS	PROTEIN	FAT	CALS
CALORIES CONSUMED					

Muscle Mastery 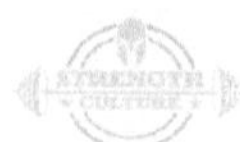

DATE: __________________

M   T   W   T   F   S   S

DAILY STEPS: __________________

DAILY GOALS : __________________

MUSCLE GROUP : __________________

TOTAL TIME: __________________

EXERCISE LOG

	EXERCISE	Sets	Reps	Intensity	1ST SET	2ND SET	3RD SET	4TH SET	5TH SET	REST
1										
2										
3										
4										
5										
6										
7										
8										
9										
10										

MOOD AND ENERGY LEVELS

CARDIO

TYPE	TIME	CALORIES BURNED'

NUTRITION TRACKER

BODY WEIGHT: _______________________________

BODY FAT %: _______________________________

SLEEP (HOURS): _______________________________

SUPPLEMENTS: _______________________________

Water

FOOD/MEAL	SERV	CARBS	PROTEIN	FAT	CALS
CALORIES CONSUMED					

Muscle Mastery

DATE: [________]

M T W T F S S

DAILY STEPS: ___________

MUSCLE GROUP: ___________

DAILY GOALS: ___________

TOTAL TIME: ___________

EXERCISE LOG

	EXERCISE	Sets	Reps	Intensity	1ST SET	2ND SET	3RD SET	4TH SET	5TH SET	REST
1										
2										
3										
4										
5										
6										
7										
8										
9										
10										

MOOD AND ENERGY LEVELS

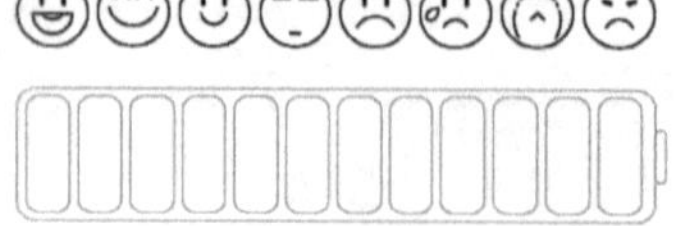

CARDIO

TYPE	TIME	CALORIES BURNED'

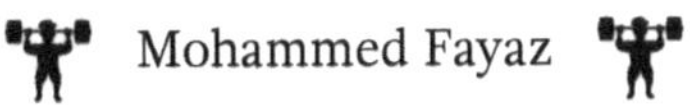

NUTRITION TRACKER

BODY WEIGHT: _______________________________

BODY FAT %: _______________________________

SLEEP (HOURS): _______________________________

SUPPLEMENTS: _______________________________

Water

FOOD/MEAL	SERV	CARBS	PROTEIN	FAT	CALS
CALORIES CONSUMED					

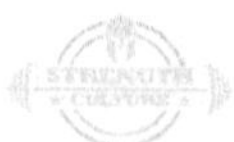 Muscle Mastery

DATE: __________

M   T   W   T   F   S   S

DAILY STEPS: __________   **MUSCLE GROUP:** __________

DAILY GOALS: __________   **TOTAL TIME:** __________

EXERCISE LOG

	EXERCISE	Sets	Reps	Intensity	1ST SET	2ND SET	3RD SET	4TH SET	5TH SET	REST
1										
2										
3										
4										
5										
6										
7										
8										
9										
10										

MOOD AND ENERGY LEVELS

CARDIO

TYPE	TIME	CALORIES BURNED'

NUTRITION TRACKER

BODY WEIGHT: ______________________________

BODY FAT %: ______________________________

SLEEP (HOURS): ______________________________

SUPPLEMENTS: ______________________________

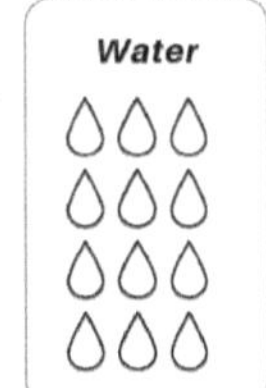

FOOD/MEAL	SERV	CARBS	PROTEIN	FAT	CALS
CALORIES CONSUMED					

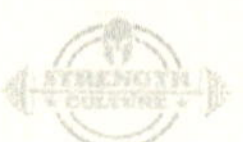 Muscle Mastery

DATE: [ ]

M T W T F S S

DAILY STEPS: __________

MUSCLE GROUP: __________

DAILY GOALS: __________

TOTAL TIME: __________

EXERCISE LOG

	EXERCISE	Sets	Reps	Intensity	1ST SET	2ND SET	3RD SET	4TH SET	5TH SET	REST
1										
2										
3										
4										
5										
6										
7										
8										
9										
10										

MOOD AND ENERGY LEVELS

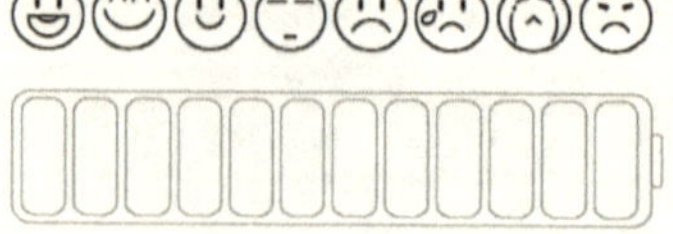

CARDIO

TYPE	TIME	CALORIES BURNED'

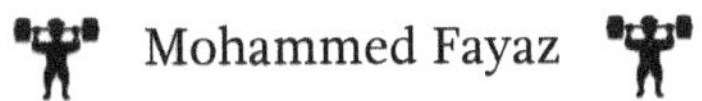 Mohammed Fayaz

NUTRITION TRACKER

BODY WEIGHT: _______________________

BODY FAT %: _______________________

SLEEP (HOURS): _______________________

SUPPLEMENTS: _______________________

Water

FOOD/MEAL	SERV	CARBS	PROTEIN	FAT	CALS
CALORIES CONSUMED					

Muscle Mastery 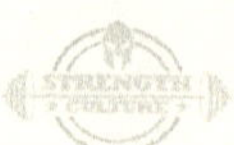

DATE: [_______________]

M T W T F S S

DAILY STEPS: _______________   **MUSCLE GROUP :** _______________

DAILY GOALS : _______________   **TOTAL TIME:** _______________

EXERCISE LOG

	EXERCISE	Sets	Reps	Intensity	1ST SET	2ND SET	3RD SET	4TH SET	5TH SET	REST
1										
2										
3										
4										
5										
6										
7										
8										
9										
10										

MOOD AND ENERGY LEVELS

CARDIO

TYPE	TIME	CALORIES BURNED'

NUTRITION TRACKER

BODY WEIGHT: _______________________________

BODY FAT %: _______________________________

SLEEP (HOURS): _______________________________

SUPPLEMENTS: _______________________________

Water

FOOD/MEAL	SERV	CARBS	PROTEIN	FAT	CALS
CALORIES CONSUMED					

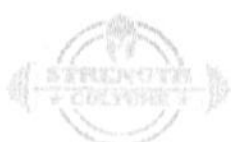 Muscle Mastery

DATE: [____________]

M T W T F S S

DAILY STEPS: ___________________   **MUSCLE GROUP :** ___________

DAILY GOALS : ___________________   **TOTAL TIME:** ___________

EXERCISE LOG

	EXERCISE	Sets	Reps	Intensity	1ST SET	2ND SET	3RD SET	4TH SET	5TH SET	REST
1										
2										
3										
4										
5										
6										
7										
8										
9										
10										

MOOD AND ENERGY LEVELS

CARDIO

TYPE	TIME	CALORIES BURNED'

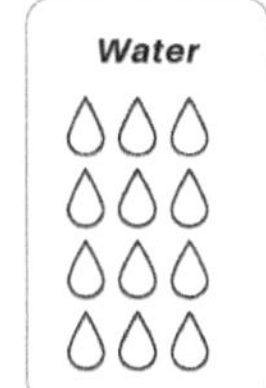

Mohammed Fayaz

NUTRITION TRACKER

BODY WEIGHT: _______________________________

BODY FAT %: _______________________________

SLEEP (HOURS): _______________________________

SUPPLEMENTS: _______________________________

Water

FOOD/MEAL	SERV	CARBS	PROTEIN	FAT	CALS
CALORIES CONSUMED					

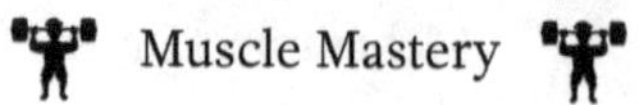 # Muscle Mastery 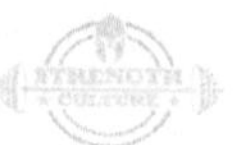

DATE: __________________

M   T   W   T   F   S   S

DAILY STEPS: __________________   **MUSCLE GROUP :** __________________

DAILY GOALS : __________________   **TOTAL TIME:** __________________

EXERCISE LOG

	EXERCISE	Sets	Reps	Intensity	1ST SET	2ND SET	3RD SET	4TH SET	5TH SET	REST
1										
2										
3										
4										
5										
6										
7										
8										
9										
10										

MOOD AND ENERGY LEVELS

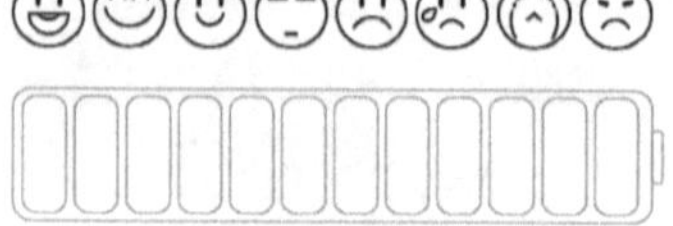

CARDIO

TYPE	TIME	CALORIES BURNED'

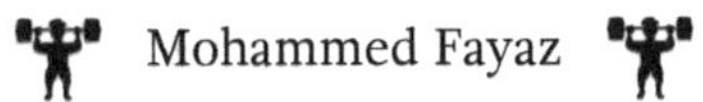

NUTRITION TRACKER

BODY WEIGHT: _______________________

BODY FAT %: _______________________

SLEEP (HOURS): _______________________

SUPPLEMENTS: _______________________

Water

FOOD/MEAL	SERV	CARBS	PROTEIN	FAT	CALS
CALORIES CONSUMED					

Muscle Mastery

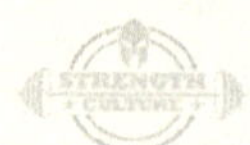

DATE: [____________]

M   T   W   T   F   S   S

DAILY STEPS: ______________

MUSCLE GROUP: ______________

DAILY GOALS: ______________

TOTAL TIME: ______________

EXERCISE LOG

	EXERCISE	Sets	Reps	Intensity	1ST SET	2ND SET	3RD SET	4TH SET	5TH SET	REST
1										
2										
3										
4										
5										
6										
7										
8										
9										
10										

MOOD AND ENERGY LEVELS

CARDIO

TYPE	TIME	CALORIES BURNED'

NUTRITION TRACKER

BODY WEIGHT: _______________________________

BODY FAT %: _______________________________

SLEEP (HOURS): _______________________________

SUPPLEMENTS: _______________________________

Water

FOOD/MEAL	SERV	CARBS	PROTEIN	FAT	CALS
CALORIES CONSUMED					

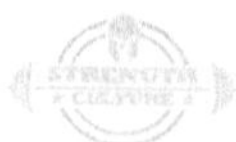 **Muscle Mastery**

DATE: __________
M   T   W   T   F   S   S

DAILY STEPS: __________

MUSCLE GROUP: __________

DAILY GOALS: __________

TOTAL TIME: __________

EXERCISE LOG

	EXERCISE	Sets	Reps	Intensity	1ST SET	2ND SET	3RD SET	4TH SET	5TH SET	REST
1										
2										
3										
4										
5										
6										
7										
8										
9										
10										

MOOD AND ENERGY LEVELS

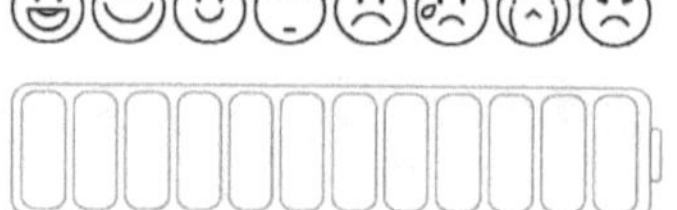

CARDIO

TYPE	TIME	CALORIES BURNED'

NUTRITION TRACKER

BODY WEIGHT: _______________________

BODY FAT %: _______________________

SLEEP (HOURS): _______________________

SUPPLEMENTS: _______________________

Water

FOOD/MEAL	SERV	CARBS	PROTEIN	FAT	CALS
CALORIES CONSUMED					

Muscle Mastery 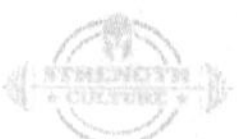

DATE:

M   T   W   T   F   S   S

DAILY STEPS:

MUSCLE GROUP :

DAILY GOALS :

TOTAL TIME:

EXERCISE LOG

	EXERCISE	Sets	Reps	Intensity	1ST SET	2ND SET	3RD SET	4TH SET	5TH SET	REST
1										
2										
3										
4										
5										
6										
7										
8										
9										
10										

MOOD AND ENERGY LEVELS

CARDIO

TYPE	TIME	CALORIES BURNED'

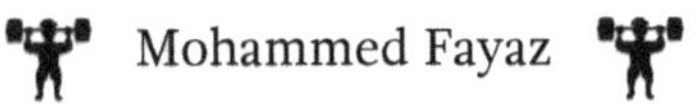

NUTRITION TRACKER

BODY WEIGHT: _______________________

BODY FAT %: _______________________

SLEEP (HOURS): _______________________

SUPPLEMENTS: _______________________

Water

FOOD/MEAL	SERV	CARBS	PROTEIN	FAT	CALS
CALORIES CONSUMED					

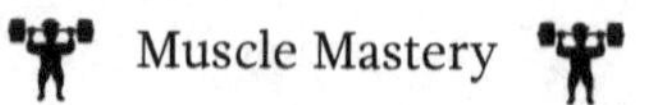

Muscle Mastery

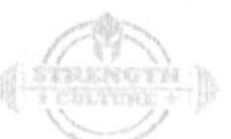

DATE: [_______________]

M   T   W   T   F   S   S

DAILY STEPS: _______________

MUSCLE GROUP: _______________

DAILY GOALS: _______________

TOTAL TIME: _______________

EXERCISE LOG

	EXERCISE	Sets	Reps	Intensity	1ST SET	2ND SET	3RD SET	4TH SET	5TH SET	REST
1										
2										
3										
4										
5										
6										
7										
8										
9										
10										

MOOD AND ENERGY LEVELS

CARDIO

TYPE	TIME	CALORIES BURNED'

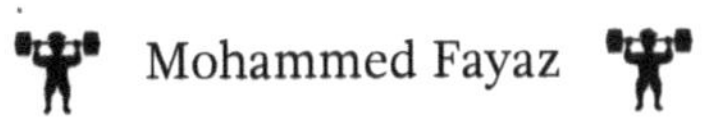

NUTRITION TRACKER

BODY WEIGHT: _______________________

BODY FAT %: _______________________

SLEEP (HOURS): _______________________

SUPPLEMENTS: _______________________

Water

FOOD/MEAL	SERV	CARBS	PROTEIN	FAT	CALS
CALORIES CONSUMED					

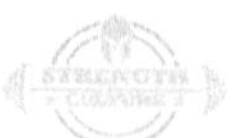

Muscle Mastery

DATE: ____________________

M T W T F S S

DAILY STEPS: __________________

MUSCLE GROUP: __________________

DAILY GOALS: __________________

TOTAL TIME: __________________

EXERCISE LOG

	EXERCISE	Sets	Reps	Intensity	1ST SET	2ND SET	3RD SET	4TH SET	5TH SET	REST
1										
2										
3										
4										
5										
6										
7										
8										
9										
10										

MOOD AND ENERGY LEVELS

CARDIO

TYPE	TIME	CALORIES BURNED'

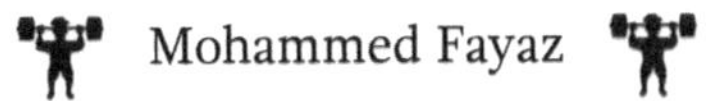

NUTRITION TRACKER

BODY WEIGHT: _______________________

BODY FAT %: _______________________

SLEEP (HOURS): _______________________

SUPPLEMENTS: _______________________

Water

FOOD/MEAL	SERV	CARBS	PROTEIN	FAT	CALS
CALORIES CONSUMED					

Muscle Mastery

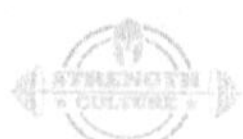

DATE:

M   T   W   T   F   S   S

DAILY STEPS:

DAILY GOALS:

MUSCLE GROUP:

TOTAL TIME:

EXERCISE LOG

	EXERCISE	Sets	Reps	Intensity	1ST SET	2ND SET	3RD SET	4TH SET	5TH SET	REST
1										
2										
3										
4										
5										
6										
7										
8										
9										
10										

MOOD AND ENERGY LEVELS

CARDIO

TYPE	TIME	CALORIES BURNED'

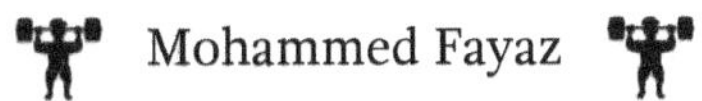

NUTRITION TRACKER

BODY WEIGHT: ___________________

BODY FAT %: ___________________

SLEEP (HOURS): ___________________

SUPPLEMENTS: ___________________

Water

FOOD/MEAL	SERV	CARBS	PROTEIN	FAT	CALS
CALORIES CONSUMED					

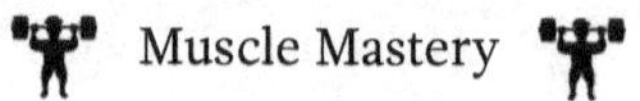 # Muscle Mastery 

DATE: [　　　　　　　　]

M T W T F S S

DAILY STEPS: ______________

MUSCLE GROUP : ______________

DAILY GOALS : ______________

TOTAL TIME: ______________

EXERCISE LOG

	EXERCISE	Sets	Reps	Intensity	1ST SET	2ND SET	3RD SET	4TH SET	5TH SET	REST
1										
2										
3										
4										
5										
6										
7										
8										
9										
10										

MOOD AND ENERGY LEVELS

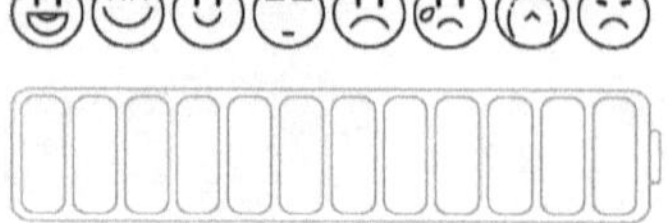

CARDIO

TYPE	TIME	CALORIES BURNED'

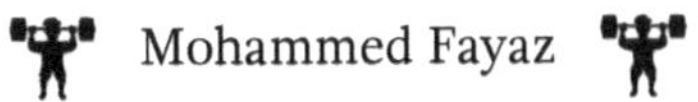

NUTRITION TRACKER

BODY WEIGHT: _______________________

BODY FAT %: _______________________

SLEEP (HOURS): _______________________

SUPPLEMENTS: _______________________

Water

FOOD/MEAL	SERV	CARBS	PROTEIN	FAT	CALS
CALORIES CONSUMED					

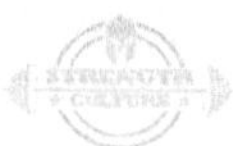 Muscle Mastery

DATE: [   ]

M   T   W   T   F   S   S

DAILY STEPS: ______________________   **MUSCLE GROUP :** ______________________

DAILY GOALS : ______________________   **TOTAL TIME:** ______________________

EXERCISE LOG

	EXERCISE	Sets	Reps	Intensity	1ST SET	2ND SET	3RD SET	4TH SET	5TH SET	REST
1										
2										
3										
4										
5										
6										
7										
8										
9										
10										

MOOD AND ENERGY LEVELS

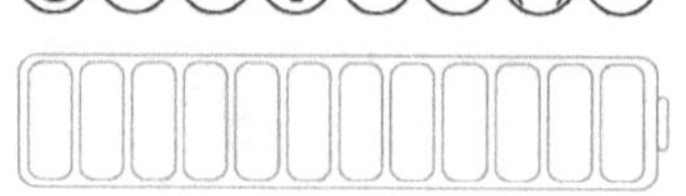

CARDIO

TYPE	TIME	CALORIES BURNED'

NUTRITION TRACKER

BODY WEIGHT: _______________________

BODY FAT %: _______________________

SLEEP (HOURS): _______________________

SUPPLEMENTS: _______________________

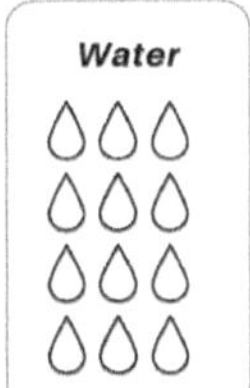

FOOD/MEAL	SERV	CARBS	PROTEIN	FAT	CALS
CALORIES CONSUMED					

Muscle Mastery 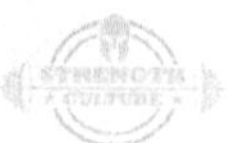

DATE: __________

M T W T F S S

DAILY STEPS: __________   **MUSCLE GROUP:** __________

DAILY GOALS: __________   **TOTAL TIME:** __________

EXERCISE LOG

	EXERCISE	Sets	Reps	Intensity	1ST SET	2ND SET	3RD SET	4TH SET	5TH SET	REST
1										
2										
3										
4										
5										
6										
7										
8										
9										
10										

MOOD AND ENERGY LEVELS

CARDIO

TYPE	TIME	CALORIES BURNED'

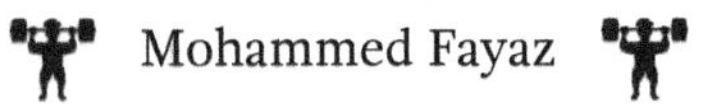

NUTRITION TRACKER

BODY WEIGHT: ___________________________

BODY FAT %: ___________________________

SLEEP (HOURS): ___________________________

SUPPLEMENTS: ___________________________

Water

FOOD/MEAL	SERV	CARBS	PROTEIN	FAT	CALS
CALORIES CONSUMED					

Muscle Mastery

MONTHLY
REFLECTION
Journal

DATE: TIME:

✦ **Monthly Wins**

✦ **How does it make me feel?**

____

____

✦ **Challenges**

✦ **How can I improve it?**

____

____

Accomplished Goals   **Unaccomplished Goals**   **Goals Next Month**

Habits Retained   **Habits Eliminated**   **New Habits Developed**
(Good & Bad)

Three things that I am most grateful for this month:

Two life lessons I learned this month:

One word that best describes this month:

How will you rate this month?   ☆☆☆☆☆

Exercise Program

SCAN THIS QR CODE TO DOWNLOAD 24 WEEKS EXERCISE
PROGRAM

STEP 1 – Download google sheet app before scanning the qr code.

STEP 2 – Give request access to grant permission

STEP 3 – Wait for 8-12 hours to grant permission and scan again to use the program.

STEP 4 – Please make a copy link of this program for your personal use and save it in your notes, do not share it with anyone. If any misuse is detected, your access will be removed and you will no longer be able to use the program.

STEP 5 – After accessing the program in Google Sheets, go to the top right corner and click the drop-down menu. Select "Share and export," then choose "Copy link." Save this link in your notes for future use.

STEP 6 – Please read the phase overview carefully in the sheet before running the program, Keep your log book and enter the data everyday

STEP 7 – Share with us your progress in social media by tagging us on instagram.

InstaPage – Fayaz_coach

Gym – Strength_culture

Book page – muscle_mastery_1